Heart Smart™

A PLAN FOR
LOW - CHOLESTEROL
LIVING
REVISED AND UPDATED

BY GAIL L. BECKER, R.D.

INTRODUCTION BY ARAM CHOBANIAN, M. D.

A FIRESIDE BOOK
PUBLISHED BY SIMON & SCHUSTER, INC.
New York   London   Toronto   Sydney   Tokyo   Singapore

Contributing authors:
Erica Rubinstein, M.S., R.D.
Pamela Richard
Copyright © 1984, 1987 by Merrell Dow Pharmaceuticals Inc.
All rights reserved
including the right of reproduction
in whole or in part in any form
Revised Fireside Edition, 1987
Published by Simon & Schuster, Inc.
Simon & Schuster Building
Rockefeller Center
1230 Avenue of the Americas
New York, NY 10020
FIRESIDE and colophon are registered trademarks of
Simon & Schuster, Inc.
HEART SMART™ is a trademark of Merrell Dow Pharmaceuticals Inc.
Manufactured in the United States of America
5 7 9 10 8 6
Library of Congress Cataloging in Publication Data
Becker, Gail L.
Heart smart.
"A Fireside book."
Bibliography: p.
Includes index.
1. Low cholesterol diet—Recipes. 2. Heart—Diseases
—Prevention. I. Title
RM237.75.B43   1987   641.5'6311   87-23690
ISBN 0-671-64761-X

ACKNOWLEDGMENTS

I would like to thank Aram Chobanian, M.D., director of the Cardiovascular Institute at the Boston University School of Medicine and professor of medicine at Boston University, and John Foreyt, Ph.D., director of the Diet Modification Clinic at Baylor College of Medicine, for their contributions to the preparation of this book.

Acknowledgments would not be complete without reference to Merrell Dow Pharmaceuticals Inc., whose commitment to cardiovascular health made this book possible.

I would also like to thank Elizabeth Hanna Schwartz for assistance in recipe development and testing and Bonnie Glass for assistance in performing the nutritional analyses.

C O N T E N T S

INTRODUCTION
by Aram Chobanian, M.D.

Aram Chobanian, M.D., is director of the Cardiovascular Institute at the Boston University School of Medicine and professor of medicine at Boston University.

☐ A healthy heart is usually a matter of personal choice. Most of the major causes of heart disease are preventable but, unfortunately, preventive measures are not widely practiced.

If you have been diagnosed as having atherosclerosis, or "hardening of the arteries," you are not alone.

Did you know that one of four Americans suffers from cardiovascular disease, and that, incredible as it seems, heart disease and its many complications account for as many deaths as all other diseases combined? This means that one of every two deaths can be attributed to heart disease. Atherosclerosis and resulting heart and blood vessel problems head the list. See Table A.

TABLE A
Leading Causes of Death

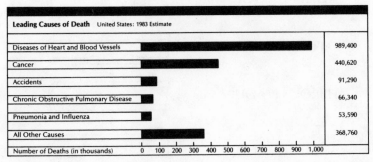

Leading Causes of Death — United States: 1983 Estimate	
Diseases of Heart and Blood Vessels	989,400
Cancer	440,620
Accidents	91,290
Chronic Obstructive Pulmonary Disease	66,340
Pneumonia and Influenza	53,590
All Other Causes	368,760
Number of Deaths (in thousands) 0 100 200 300 400 500 600 700 800 900 1,000	

SOURCE: National Center for Health Statistics, U.S. Public Health Service, DHHS. See 1986 Heart Facts: American Heart Association

If this sounds frightening, it should. If you have athero-sclerosis, the good news is there are many contributing factors within your control. The three most important factors—hypertension, high blood cholesterol and cigarette smoking (each capable of doubling or even tripling your risk of a heart attack)—can be controlled through diet, proper exercise and a successful smoking cessation program.

If the water pipes in your sink were rusty and clogged, chances are you'd repair them. In atherosclerosis, cholesterol and other fatty substances build up inside your blood vessels like the rust in old pipes and impede the flow of oxygen-rich blood to your heart. Once your vessels have been damaged by cholesterol deposits, scar tissue may form around the "injured" artery and enlarge the obstruction. The result can be severe chest pain and, eventually, heart attack.

Cholesterol is the main substance found in obstructed arteries. This is often called "plaque." Table B depicts the stages of atherosclerosis.

TABLE B
Stages of Atherosclerosis

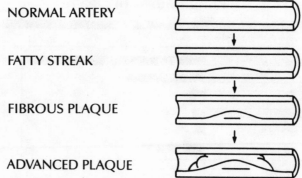

NORMAL ARTERY

FATTY STREAK

FIBROUS PLAQUE

ADVANCED PLAQUE

SOURCE: Grundy, Scott, M., M.D.; "Atherosclerosis: Pathology, Pathogenesis, and Role of Risk Factors." *Disease-A-Month,* Year Book Medical Publishers, Inc., Chicago, Illinois, 1983.

Although cholesterol is a fatty substance needed by the body to build cells and make hormones, high blood cholesterol forces the progression of atherosclerosis, increasing the chances for a heart attack or stroke.

The evidence for this relationship between high cholesterol and atherosclerosis is overwhelming. In experimental animal studies, it is virtually impossible to produce atherosclerosis without the presence of high blood cholesterol. A landmark study, referred to as the Lipid Research Clinics Coronary Primary Prevention Trial (LRC-CPPT), showed that men who reduced their blood cholesterol levels through diet in combination with cholesterol-lowering drugs had fewer heart attacks than men whose cholesterol remained elevated.[1,2]

Because cholesterol does not dissolve in blood, it must be carried in packages of fat and protein called "lipoproteins." These are manufactured in the body. Two of the most important kinds of lipoproteins are high-density lipoproteins (HDL) and low-density lipoproteins (LDL). HDL is often referred to as "good cholesterol" because it is believed to remove excess cholesterol from body tissues and carry the cholesterol away for excretion. LDL is often referred to as "bad cholesterol" because it tends to deposit cholesterol on artery walls, contributing to the development of atherosclerosis.

Higher levels of HDL cholesterol (thought to protect against heart disease) have been seen in people who exercise regularly, don't smoke and drink only moderately. Higher LDL cholesterol levels have been associated with sedentary living, obesity and diets high in saturated fats. Elevations in LDL cholesterol may also be the result of genetics. It has been shown clearly that members of families afflicted with the problem have a very high risk of premature death from heart attacks.

Your physician determines whether or not your blood cholesterol is too high by measuring your levels of total blood cholesterol, HDL and LDL cholesterol and comparing these values to established guidelines. The National Institutes of Health recently recommended cholesterol levels below 200 mg/dl.

Table C shows how your cholesterol level affects your risk of developing heart disease.

Those with borderline-high values should follow the Heart Smart plan outlined in Chapter III and recheck blood cholesterol within one year. If additional risk factors are present, or if you fall into the high blood cholesterol category, your doctor will advise a stringent Heart Smart diet plan. This group often includes individuals with genetically high cholesterol.

Both borderline-high and high-risk groups need to reduce dietary fat and cholesterol; those in the high-risk group may also need drugs to help lower cholesterol.

TABLE C
Initial Classification Based on Total Cholesterol

BLOOD CHOLESTEROL LEVEL (MG/DL)		
desirable	borderline high	high
200 or less	200–239	240 and above

SOURCE: National Cholesterol Education Program Report of the Expert Panel on Detection, Evaluation and Treatment of High Blood Cholesterol in Adults (NIH publication No. 88-2925, January 1988)

High blood cholesterol levels can be caused by heredity and the foods you eat. Foods high in saturated fat—such as animal products like meat, eggs, butter and cheese—contribute to elevated blood cholesterol levels. Some plant sources of fat—like coconut, palm and palm kernel oils—also contain saturated fats.

Some fats appear to lower blood cholesterol levels. Recent studies suggest that monounsaturated fats, such as olive oil, may have this characteristic.

Polyunsaturated fats—such as corn, safflower and sunflower oils—are also recommended as substitutes for saturated fats.

The ratio, or balance, of the types of fat you eat is important for heart health.

It is advisable to restrict your fat intake to fewer than 30 percent of the calories you consume each day, with fewer than 10 percent from saturated fats. Refer to Chapter III to learn how this fits into your personal eating plan. The ratio of polyunsaturated fats to saturated fats is called a P:S ratio and can be found on many food labels. This information can help you control the amount and type of fat you consume each day.

As you can see, a major factor within your control—your diet—can help to lower body cholesterol.

Other risk factors for heart disease are:

□ male sex
□ family history
□ cigarette smoking
□ high blood pressure (hypertension)
□ diabetes mellitus
□ obesity
□ lack of exercise

If your blood cholesterol level is high, these risk factors are even more dangerous. They act synergistically to compound the effect of each.

Smoking can more than double your risk of a heart attack. It appears somehow to damage artery walls, allowing cholesterol to accumulate faster. But if you quit, your risk of a heart attack is rapidly reduced. If you quit for at least 10 years, your risk drops to that of a non-smoker.

High blood pressure, or hypertension, speeds up atherosclerosis. It seems to damage blood vessels and thereby promotes the accumulation of cholesterol in artery walls. It is a very important risk factor and one that can be readily controlled. It is estimated that between 57 and 59 million Americans have this silent evil, but many are unaware of it.

Blood pressure is the pressure exerted by the blood against the blood vessels. A pressure of 120/80 is considered normal. The top pressure (systolic) is the peak value created when your heart contracts. The lower figure (diastolic) is the minimum value present when your heart relaxes. When blood pressure increases, your heart must work harder to circulate your blood.

High blood pressure is defined as any value greater than 140/90, much lower than the values doctors once thought were safe. There's a continual increase in the risk of cardiovascular disease as blood pressure rises above 130 for sytolic pressure and above 85 for diastolic pressure. Approximately a quarter of all American adults have blood pressure above 140/90 and, even more surprisingly, two-thirds of Americans over age 65 have blood pressure above this level.

An informed person can take steps to reduce this risk factor. First, have your blood pressure checked by a doctor or nurse. Being overweight is a contributing factor to high blood pressure. So is excessive consumption of salt. The HEART SMART™ plan discusses weight control and sodium reduction, but discuss your individual plan with a doctor. You may also need medication to lower blood pressure.

Diabetes, a disease that causes high blood sugar, is

another significant risk factor for heart disease. Although the exact reason is poorly understood, high blood sugar is associated with damage to blood vessels and acceleration of atherosclerosis. The most common type of diabetes occurs in overweight adults, and weight control, proper diet and, sometimes, medication should be used to bring blood sugar down and help delay the development of heart disease.

Obese people are more at risk for atherosclerosis than those at their desirable weight. Being overweight may produce abnormal fats in the body that contribute to heart disease. Obese people are also more likely to have additional risk factors such as hypertension and diabetes.

Lack of exercise, common in obese people, is also associated with a greater risk of heart disease. Studies show that individuals who exercise regularly have higher amounts of HDL, or "good cholesterol," than sedentary people. Elevations in HDL, accomplished through exercise, may protect against heart disease. For more on exercise, see Chapter II.

TABLE D
Heart Disease Combined Risk Factors

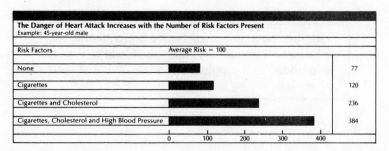

The Danger of Heart Attack Increases with the Number of Risk Factors Present Example: 45-year-old male		
Risk Factors	Average Risk = 100	
None		77
Cigarettes		120
Cigarettes and Cholesterol		236
Cigarettes, Cholesterol and High Blood Pressure		384
	0 100 200 300 400	

SOURCE: Framingham Heart Study. See 1986 Heart Facts: American Heart Association

The dangers of heart attack increase with the number of risk factors present. This chart shows how a combination of three major risk factors can increase the likelihood of heart attack. For purposes of illustration, this chart uses an abnormal blood pressure level of 180 systolic and a cholesterol level of 310 in a 45-year-old man.

These risk factors are important because they are cumulative: the more risk factors present, the greater your chances of having a heart attack. See Table D for a graphic description.

You, and only you, can decide to change risk factors within your control.

The HEART SMART™ Goals are:

□ Achieve or maintain your ideal body weight.
□ Decrease your intake of total fat.
□ Decrease saturated fat and cholesterol.
□ Decrease your intake of sodium (salt).

Your doctor may prescribe medicine to lower cholesterol or blood pressure, especially if you fall into the "high-risk" category as indicated on page 12.

In some cases, your doctor may enlist the help of a registered dietitian. But only you can follow through with the changes necessary to live a healthier life. Remember, a healthy heart may be a matter of personal choice. This book is a good place to begin.

Although no plan can guarantee better health, the information that follows may be of help to you. It is intended as a supplement to the advice of your physician.

CHAPTER 1

□

EATING FOR HEART HEALTH

□ As you start on your plan to change habits acquired over a lifetime, it's encouraging to realize you have plenty of company.

Since the early 1960s, millions of Americans have learned about the risks of atherosclerosis and coronary heart disease and have successfully changed their lifestyles.

The American Heart Association reports that since 1964 the average per capita intake of saturated fat and cholesterol has declined and, correspondingly, cholesterol levels in adults have decreased. Millions of American adults have stopped smoking.[3] Many American adults with high blood pressure are learning to reduce their intake of sodium.

As mentioned in the introduction, cholesterol is necessary to a healthy body. It acts as an insulator of nerve and brain tissue. An important part of the cell membrane, it makes your skin almost completely waterproof, while at the same time retarding evaporation of water from the body.

Since your body needs cholesterol, it ensures a supply by manufacturing it. But when a high dietary intake of cholesterol is added to your body's naturally produced cholesterol, your system may become overloaded.

Diet is the major key to reducing cholesterol and controlling atherosclerosis. A regular weight-control program, integrating diet and exercise, takes commitment. As you progressively change your habits, making your plan part of a permanent lifestyle, it becomes easier and easier until it is second nature.

The importance of diet in lowering body cholesterol can be seen in recent studies. A group of researchers at the University of Minnesota has found that vegetarian diets containing no animal fats result in lower blood cholesterol levels.[4]

In studies of Japan's population, it seems that increasing Westernization in that nation has been accompanied by an increase in death from heart disease. Compared to the U.S. population, Japanese in Japan have low cholesterol levels. However, Japanese living in California and eating American diets have relatively high cholesterol levels, and the severity of atherosclerosis approaches that of Caucasians in the United States.[5]

A recent research trial provides strong support for the role of nutrition in preventing heart disease. The study, referred to as MR. FIT (Multiple Risk Factors Intervention Trial), showed that men who experienced the greatest reductions in plasma cholesterol were those who adhered to diets lowest in total fat, saturated fat and cholesterol.[6]

Besides cholesterol and fat, other dietary factors may influence blood-cholesterol levels. Recent studies suggest that omega-3 fatty acids—a type of fat found in cold and deep-water fish such as salmon, tuna and mackerel—lower the level of harmful LDL cholesterol and may raise the level of beneficial HDL cholesterol.

Interest in the benefits of fish was sparked by the observation that Greenland Eskimos experience low rates of heart disease despite a very high dietary intake of fat.[7] The type of fat—omega-3—was the key. Subsequent studies have shown significant reductions in the incidence of heart disease when fatty fish is consumed at least twice a week.[8]

Besides lowering the levels of harmful LDL cholesterol, fatty fish may actually protect against heart attack by making blood platelets less sticky and, therefore, less likely to form clots that cause heart attacks. Fatty fish may also play a role in lowering blood pressure.

Another dietary factor in the spotlight is monounsaturated fat, of which olive and avocado are the most common. New studies suggest that these types of fats can also help lower the level of harmful LDL cholesterol.[9]

Certain forms of fiber such as "gums" and pectins—found in legumes, some fruits and vegetables, oats, oat bran and barley—also play a role in lowering blood cholesterol levels. Although poorly understood, these soluble fibers move through the small intestine and interfere with either the absorption or the metabolism of cholesterol.[10]

The good news is that Americans are becoming more aware of the relationship between diet and disease.

As a nation, we are eating more vegetables, fruit, fish and chicken and fewer animal fats such as beef and dairy products. The latter foods have been status symbols in the affluent industrial countries, which have traditionally had the highest incidence of heart disease.[11, 12, 13, 14]

Between 1963 and 1977, per capita consumption of animal fats fell almost 50 percent in America. Perhaps this accounts for the dramatic drop in heart disease among adult Americans.[15]

Modifying your eating and other lifestyle habits is discussed in Chapters II and IV. It is up to you and your doctor to determine the combination of diet and exercise that fits into your future life/health plan. In the meantime, such changes for the general public are a topic of debate among scientists.

Some researchers believe that there should be major changes in the American diet. Others think it would be premature to recommend any changes at all. A more moderate approach is taken by those who advocate individual prescription. These health professionals have concluded that evidence suggests a relationship between diet and coronary heart disease. But they agree that the risks don't apply to everyone.

Individual prescription—a diet combined with an exercise program and possible drug therapy based on a physician's judgment as to the special health needs of each patient—seems to be the most sensible approach.

We all know people who have changed their lives through diet and exercise and have adopted a missionary zeal toward converting friends who haven't yet "seen the light." The truth is, not everyone needs to change.

You, on the other hand, have been told by your doctor that you have a cholesterol level that is too high. The most exciting aspect of choosing a healthier approach is that you, yourself, can make it happen.

CHAPTER 11

□

CHANGING LIFESTYLES: EATING AND EXERCISING

BY JOHN FOREYT, PH.D.

Dr. John Foreyt is director of the Diet Modification Clinic at Baylor College of Medicine, Houston, Texas.

□ Changing a diet that you have been eating for years isn't always as simple as it may sound. Ingrained eating habits influence to a great degree just what and how much you eat.

The first step in putting a new diet plan into action is to take a look at your eating habits. Also consider why you've developed these habits. The key to success is replacing negative habits with positive behavior.

The main reason so many diet and exercise weight-control programs fail is that people often think of them as a temporary inconvenience, a necessary evil designed to take off weight by the wedding, before summer, by the holidays. When the diet is over, it's back to the same old eating patterns that caused all the trouble in the first place.

Doctors agree that the only way to take weight off and keep it off is to make basic lifestyle changes. At the Diet Modification Clinic at Baylor College of Medicine in Houston, Texas, we teach patients to do this through a process called behavior modification: changing your behavior patterns and long-standing eating habits.

We have devised a plan to teach people how to take control of their eating habits. After two months of behavior-modification sessions aimed at changing eating behavior, about three-quarters of the overweight patients were able to maintain their weight loss or continue to lose. Our studies have followed these patients up to a year. In this chapter, we will share with you many of the tips included in the Baylor program to aid you in making positive changes in your behavior.

HOW TO BEGIN

With your doctor, select a good diet—one low in cholesterol, saturated fat and sodium—like the HEART SMART Diet outlined in Chapter III. Then begin your behavior-modification program as outlined below so that you can incorporate your diet plan into your life plan.

THE DIETARY DETECTIVE

To change your eating habits, you must first identify them. Each day write everything you eat and drink in a small notebook, or photocopy the Food Record Sheet at the end of this chapter (Table IIC) and use it to keep a complete record of everything that goes into your mouth. This means not just at mealtime, but all the time. Don't forget that bite of tuna you took while you were making sandwiches. Or the tasting you did to make sure the stew was seasoned just right. Or the three crackers you grabbed after you came in the door tonight just to "tide you over" until dinner. Note the time of day you had the food, where you ate, your mood when you ate each item and with whom you ate. If you are dieting to lose pounds, keep a record of your weight. Hang a sheet of graph paper near the scale, and weigh yourself each day at the same time, noting your own ups and downs (see sample in Table IIA). The numbers on the vertical axis should range from your present weight to your goal weight in intervals of one to five pounds.

After two weeks, study your food records to see which habits can coexist with your new diet and which need changing. Look for patterns. Find foods not permitted on your low-cholesterol, low-saturated fat, reduced-sodium eating plan.

Once you've identified self-defeating habits that have become part of your behavior, you're well on the way to changing those habits.

DELIBERATE DETOURS AND PINK PIGS

Your next step is to find ways to change your environment. If you regularly stop at a neighborhood deli on your way to work to pick up a Danish and coffee, take a different route to the office and thus avoid the impulse to stop. Don't keep off-limits snacks in the house. If another family member wants them, he or she will have to get them somewhere else.

Put notes to yourself on the mirror or refrigerator with the notation: "Those who indulge bulge." I have one patient who has decorated her refrigerator door with pink

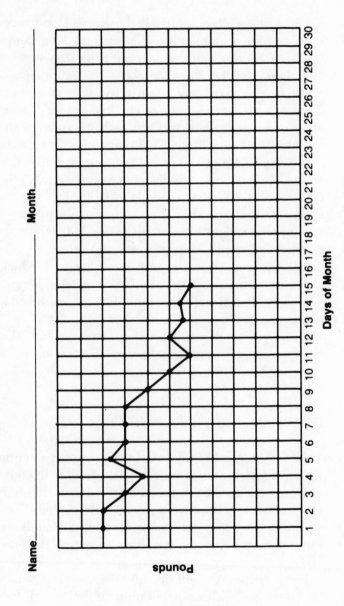

TABLE IIA
Daily Weight Record

Name

Month

Pounds

Days of Month

pig magnets that say, "You back again?" and "I'm getting thin s l o w l y."

Choose one place to eat when you're at home, and eat every meal there. Devote your entire attention to eating. This means no phone calls, television, letter writing or reading. Never eat standing up. Eliminate food cues by removing anything from your environment that causes you to eat what you shouldn't. Some examples are television commercials that present an opportunity to get a snack, office birthday cakes, certain times of day that signal snack time and other persons eating near you.

THE STRATEGIC PLANNER

Use various strategies to control your eating habits. One of these might be writing a contract with yourself. If you lose two pounds this week, you'll treat yourself to that movie you've been wanting to see. Or buy a new shirt. Or have your hair done. You can also make a pact with your spouse or a friend. One woman's husband promised to take her on a world cruise if she'd lose thirty pounds. She did, and they went. Most of us can't afford round-the-world trips, but we can afford breakfast in bed, new clothes, books or records. Make it fun—something nice you can anticipate.

Another effective strategy can take the form of stress reduction. In recording your moods, you may find that you're experiencing stress, boredom, loneliness, hostility or other negative emotions in conjunction with food binges.

To ease stress, use a relaxation technique. Sit back, close your eyes, and focus on a pleasant scene, excluding anything else from your thoughts. Stay this way for five minutes. Whenever you feel stressed, take a personal timeout. Go someplace quiet, whether it's your bedroom or the lounge at work and use this technique.

When you have negative feelings that are leading you to eat, substitute another pleasurable activity for eating. Telephone a friend. Take a relaxing bath. One patient reported that not only was her diet a great success, but she was also squeaky clean.

If you feel bored or lonely, get out and join a fitness class, a church group or any activity you can share with others.

Modeling is another strategy to help you attain your goal of continuing good health. Seek out persons who have been successful in staying on a low-cholesterol, low-saturated fat, reduced-sodium diet and use them as models. Avoid, whenever possible, persons to whom a social occasion is an excuse to "pig out."

EXERCISE YOUR WAY TO HEALTH

Exercise is a vital companion activity to any dieting program. It serves the threefold purpose of:

□ Burning calories
□ Improving muscle tone (fighting flab)
□ Improving the efficiency of your cardiovascular system

Before starting any exercise program, check with your doctor. With his or her permission, begin a regular daily program of exercise. Any aerobic exercise—such as walking, cycling or jogging—that causes the heart to beat faster than its normal rate for a sustained period—more than twenty minutes—is good. Not only does it burn calories while you're exercising, but its benefits last for hours after the exercising has stopped. Following your exercise period, your metabolic rate stays more rapid than usual for up to six hours, burning calories more efficiently for an extended period of time. Table IIB provides a more detailed list of calories burned for various forms of physical activity.

TABLE IIB
Energy Expenditure Chart

Activity	Approximate Number of Calories Used Per Hour
Lying down or sleeping	80
Sitting	100
Driving a car	120
Standing	140
Domestic work	180
Walking, 2½ mph	210
Bicycling, 5½ mph	210
Gardening	220
Golf, mowing the lawn	250
Bowling	270
Walking, 3¾ mph	300
Swimming, ½ mph	300
Square dancing, volleyball, roller skating	350
Wood chopping	400
Tennis	420
Skiing, 10 mph	600
Squash or handball	600
Bicycling, 13 mph	660
Running, 10 mph	900

Source: Figures are for a 150-pound person and are based on material prepared by Robert E. Johnson, M.D., Ph.D., and colleagues, University of Illinois.

WALKING FOR HEALTH

The most accessible, easiest and least expensive means of aerobic exercise is fast walking. Walking is also easy on the body, avoiding the shock to the bones and joints experienced in activities like jogging. And walking can be done just outside your home, without any special equipment or clothing. Walking at a good clip can burn about six calories a minute.

After a checkup by your doctor, start walking briskly about 15 minutes a day, three days a week. Gradually build this up to 45 minutes a day, three or four days a week. If you set aside a specific time each day, you'll be forming another good habit on the road to improved health and fitness.

SUCCESS IN THE LONG RUN

As you follow your diet and exercise plan, eating should be less important to you as a source of pleasure and satisfaction. For those times when you may overindulge, such as holidays and on vacations, lose weight before, not afterwards. The old excuse about eating today and dieting tomorrow is a delusion. Believe it and you will be fighting excess weight again.

If you have dropped several pounds, don't keep those baggy clothes around. Indulge in a little vanity. Buy some flattering new outfits for the slimmer you. Participate in activities you've always thought you would like: bowl, swim, exercise, cycle. Try new hobbies and activities. Enjoy the variety your new lifestyle has opened up for you.

TABLE IIC
Food Record

Name _____ **Date** _____

Time/Place	Emotion/With Whom	Food, Preparation and Amount	Food Group

CHAPTER III

□

THE HEART
SMART PLAN

□ Now that you know how to modify your eating habits and other lifestyle behaviors in order to better your health, let's talk about a special diet that can help reduce the risk of heart disease.

Too few people realize or consider that the food we eat today affects our health in both the long and the short run, today and tomorrow. As you have already learned, many of the components of foods have an impact upon the development of atherosclerosis, the precursor of coronary heart or artery disease. Too much cholesterol, saturated fat and sodium in our diets can increase our chances of developing heart disease. If obesity occurs in conjunction with high cholesterol levels, smoking or hypertension, coronary heart disease risk is significantly increased. Additionally, excessive consumption of alcohol can contribute to hypertension and increase your chances of developing heart disease. Table IIIA graphically compares the percentages of cholesterol and fat in the typical American diet versus that in the HEART SMART Plan.

A diet that controls the amount of fat, cholesterol, sodium and calories can help reduce the risk of developing coronary heart disease. In order to reduce the amount of saturated fat and cholesterol in your diet, decrease the amount of animal products you eat—such as eggs, whole milk, cheese, beef, pork and organ meats—as well as fats and oils. Such changes will also help control calories. However, if you do not need to lose weight, you should increase your intake of complex carbohydrates—such as vegetables, fruits, grains and legumes—to make up for significant decreases in calories. These foods, as mentioned in Chapter I, contain heart-healthy fiber that may lower your blood cholesterol.

TABLE IIIA

Comparison of Cholesterol and Fat in the HEART SMART Plan and the Typical American Diet

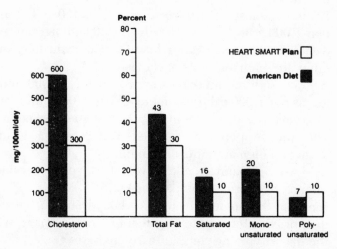

SOURCE: *Dietary Goals for the United States,* prepared by the U.S. Senate Select Committee on Nutrition and Human Needs, 1977.

Note: These values are the "upper limit" of recommendations, see diet plan.

Oftentimes a reduced sodium intake necessitates an increased potassium intake. Potassium, however, occurs in many foods, particularly vegetables, fruits, dried beans, dried peas, lentils and nuts. Getting enough potassium should not be a problem as long as you eat a well-balanced, varied diet, such as the one recommended in the HEART SMART Plan.

The HEART SMART Plan is based on the following guidelines from the American Heart Association for helping to reduce the risk of heart disease.[16]

1. Reduce total fat calories to less than 30 percent of your total caloric intake, with less than 10 percent from saturated fats, less than 10 percent from polyunsaturated fats and the remainder from monounsaturated fats. (See Appendix B for the types of fats in food products.)

2. Reduce cholesterol intake to less than 100 milligrams per 1,000 calories, not to exceed 300 milligrams per day. (See Appendix A for foods that contain low, medium and high amounts of cholesterol.)

3. Reduce sodium intake to approximately 1,000 milligrams per 1,000 calories, not to exceed 3,000 milligrams (3 grams) per day (roughly equivalent to 1 teaspoon of salt). (See Appendix C for foods that contain low, medium and high amounts of sodium.)

4. Achieve or maintain ideal weight via proper caloric intake. (See formula on pages 44 and 45.)

5. Increase the amount of total carbohydrates in the diet to approximately 50 to 55 percent of total calories, with the majority being complex carbohydrates.

6. Although not recommended, if alcoholic beverages are consumed, the caloric intake from this source should be limited to 15 percent of total calories but should not exceed 50 milliliters (about 2 ounces) of alcohol per day.

TABLE IIIB
Percent of Calories from Nutrients

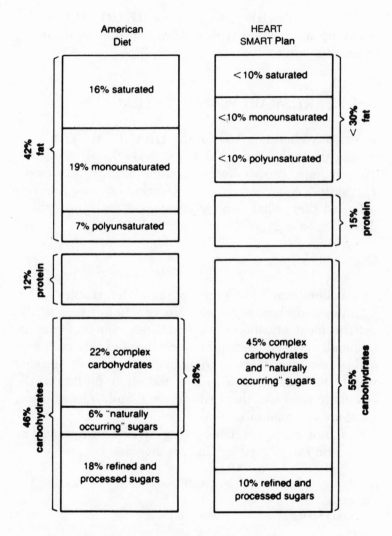

SOURCE: *Dietary Goals for the United States,* prepared by the U.S. Senate Select Committee on Nutrition and Human Needs, 1977.

This translates into 8 ounces of wine, two beers or two 1-ounce shots of whisky.

Refer to Table IIIB to see how the HEART SMART Plan stacks up against the typical American diet in regard to these guidelines.

THE HEART SMART PLAN FOOD GROUPS

To simplify choosing foods in the HEART SMART Plan, a system of food groups has been devised, based on the carbohydrate, protein and fat content of individual foods. This system is devised by nutritionists to ensure a properly balanced diet. First familiarize yourself with the groups, then use the suggested plans on pages 49–56.

VEGETABLES

As excellent sources of vitamins, minerals, complex carbohydrates and fiber, vegetables are vital to heart health. To get the most nutrition from vegetables, eat them raw or minimally cooked (steamed). Keep in mind that each vegetable provides different vitamins and minerals, making variety important. As a rule, if the outer portion of the vegetable is edible, that's where you'll find the majority of vitamins and minerals.

One unit in the vegetable group equals ½ cup cooked or 1 medium raw vegetable. Choices include:

artichoke   cabbage**
asparagus**   carrot*
bamboo shoots   cauliflower
beets   celery
broccoli***   cucumber
Brussels sprouts   eggplant

greens***(collard, endive,   scallions
   escarole, lettuce, spinach)   shallots
kohlrabi   squash*
leeks   snow peas
mushrooms   string beans
okra   sweet potatoes*
onion   tomato**
parsnip   tomato juice or tomato-juice
peas   cocktail, low-sodium
peppers***   turnips**
pumpkin*   water chestnuts
radish   yams*
rutabaga   zucchini

*Good source of vitamin A
** Good source of vitamin C
*** Good source of vitamins A and C
Note: Starchy vegetables higher in complex carbohydrates are found in the grains group. Tomato juice and tomato-juice cocktail are high in sodium. Select the low-salt variety or make your own!

FRUITS

As with vegetables, some fruits are good sources of many nutrients, including carbohydrates and fiber. In addition, fruits, unlike most desserts, can satisfy your sweet tooth without tipping the scales. Also unlike many desserts, fruits provide our bodies with a variety of important vitamins and minerals. Right column indicates unit amount for each. Choices include:

apple, fresh   □ 1 small
  juice   □ ⅓ cup
  sauce   □ ½ cup
apricots,* fresh   □ 2 medium
  canned in juice   □ 2 medium
  dried   □ 4 halves

banana	□ ½ small
berries,** except strawberries	□ ½ cup
strawberries	□ ¾ cup
cherries	□ 10 large
dates	□ 2
figs, fresh and dried	□ 2 large
fruit cocktail, fresh or canned	□ ½ cup
grapefruit,** fresh	□ ½ small
canned in juice	□ ½ cup
juice	□ ½ cup
grapes	□ 15 medium
kiwi**	□ 1 medium
kumquats	□ 4 medium
mango	□ ½ small
melon,*** except watermelon	□ ½ cup
watermelon	□ 1 cup
nectarine***	□ 1 medium
orange,** fresh	□ 1 small
Mandarin sections	□ ½ cup
juice	□ ½ cup
papaya	□ ½ cup
peach,* fresh	□ 1 medium
canned in juice	□ ½ cup
pear, fresh	□ 1 small
canned in juice	□ ½ cup
persimmon	□ 1 medium
pineapple, fresh	□ 2 slices or ½ cup
canned in juice	□ 2 slices or ½ cup
juice	□ ½ cup
plums	□ 2 medium
prunes	□ 2 medium
prune juice	□ ¼ cup
raisins	□ 2 tablespoons
tangerine**	□ 1 large

* Good source of vitamin A
** Good source of vitamin C
*** Good source of vitamins A and C

GRAINS

Foods in this group are excellent sources of complex carbohydrates, making grains important for heart health. In
addition, most grain products are excellent sources of B
vitamins and iron, and whole-grain products are good
sources of fiber. Remember, unlike wheat and other grains,
oats contain soluble fibers that may help to lower harmful
LDL-cholesterol levels. Choices include:

BREADS

bagel	□ ½ small
biscuit*	□ 1 small
bread, sandwich	□ 1 slice
cornbread, 2-inch square*	□ 1
English muffin	□ ½
muffin	□ 1 medium
roll, dinner	□ 1 small
frankfurter	□ ½
hamburger	□ ½
hard	□ ½ medium
tortilla, corn, 6-inch	□ 1
pita pocket	□ 1 small

* Omit 1 fat-group unit
All values are for products without added salt or fat.

CEREALS & PASTAS

barley, corn, oats, rice,	
wheat cereals, cold	□ 1 ounce or ¾ cup
hot, cooked	□ ½ cup
uncooked	□ ¼ cup
bran cereal	□ ⅓ cup
oat bran	□ ½ cup

pasta or noodles, cooked	□ ½ cup
wheat germ	□ ¼ cup
whole-grain kernels	
barley, buckwheat groats,	
bulgur, grits, hominy,	
rice, cooked	□ ½ cup
popcorn, air-popped	□ 2 cups

CRACKERS*

arrowroot	□ 3
breadsticks, 5 inches long, ½-	
inch wide	□ 3
flatbread, thin wafers	□ 4
graham, 2 ½-inch squares	□ 2
melba toast, rectangular	□ 5
round	□ 6
oyster	□ 20
whole-grain, 2 by 3½-inches	□ 3

* Note: Choose crackers without salt on top.

BAKING INGREDIENTS

arrowroot	□ 2 tablespoons
bread crumbs, dry, salt-free	□ 3 tablespoons
cornmeal	□ 2 tablespoons
cornstarch	□ 2 tablespoons
flour	□ 2 tablespoons
tapioca	□ 2 tablespoons

VEGETABLES

corn, whole-kernel	□ ⅓ cup
on cob	□ 1 small
peas, green	□ ½ cup
potato, white, whole	□ 1 small
mashed	□ ½ cup

squash, winter	□ ¾ cup
sweet potato (yam), whole	□ ½ small
mashed	□ ¼ cup

LEGUMES

Legumes are good sources of protein, yet contain virtually no cholesterol or fat. At the same time, they provide an abundance of complex carbohydrates, soluble fiber, vitamins and minerals. Due to their HEART SMART characteristics, legumes should be liberally included in the diet. Choices include:

DRIED BEANS (COOKED)   □ ½ cup

black	mung
Great Northern	navy
kidney	pinto
lima	white

DRIED PEAS   □ ½ cup

black-eyed
chick (garbanzo)
cow
split

LENTILS   □ ½ cup

MEAT AND ALTERNATIVES

Besides providing substantial amounts of protein, this group contributes B vitamins, iron and phosphorus to your diet. Since most animal products are high in cholesterol and saturated fat, use the purchasing and cooking tips in

Chapter IV—along with Appendices A, B, C and D—to assist you in making HEART SMART food decisions.

Accordingly, meat and alternatives are classified according to fat content. Choices include:

VERY LOW-FAT

chicken, without skin	□ 1 ounce
Cornish hen, without skin	□ 1 ounce
cottage cheese, dry	□ ¼ cup
egg whites	□ 2
fish: bass, bluefish, carp, cod, flounder, halibut, smelt, sole, whiting	□ 1 ounce
pheasant, without skin	□ 1 ounce
*tuna, packed in water	□ 1 ounce
turkey, without skin	□ 1 ounce
shellfish	
clams, shrimp, oyster	□ 5 small
lobster	□ 1 ounce
veal: cutlets, leg, loin, rib, shank, shoulder	□ 1 ounce
venison	□ 1 ounce

MODERATELY LOW-FAT

beef: chipped, flank steak, tenderloin	□ 1 ounce
**cheese:	
with less than 5 percent animal fat ***	□ 1 ounce
cottage cheese, creamed	□ ¼ cup
mozzarella, part-skim	□ 1 ounce
Parmesan (high in sodium)	□ 3 tablespoons
duck, without skin	□ 1 ounce
****fish: herring, mackerel, red snapper, salmon, sardines, swordfish, trout, tuna, whitefish	□ 1 ounce
lamb: leg, rib, roast, shank	□ 1 ounce

pork: leg, shoulder, tenderloin	□ 1 ounce
tofu	□ 3 ounces
*tuna, packed in oil	□ 1 ounce

*Choose low-sodium canned fish or rinse and drain before using.
**Cheeses are naturally high in sodium; look for the no-salt-added or low-sodium varieties.
***To calculate the percentage of fat in one serving (1 ounce or 28 grams), use the information on the product label and divide grams of fat in 1 serving (1 ounce) by 28 grams, then multiply by 100. For example: 7 grams fat/serving divided by 28 grams = .25; .25 x 100 = 25% fat content.
****Note: Fish containing high amounts of omega-3 fatty acids, such as salmon, trout, tuna and mackerel, are recommended at least two times per week for their heart-healthy characteristics. See Appendix D for additional choices.

MILK PRODUCTS

In addition to legumes and meat and alternatives, milk products are good sources of protein. However, unlike legumes and like meat and alternatives, some milk products are high in saturated fat. For this reason, choose low-fat milk products for heart health.

Most milk products are excellent sources of calcium, a nutrient important for the development and maintenance of strong bones and teeth at *all* ages. Fortified milk is also a good source of vitamins A and D. Choices include:

VERY LOW-FAT

buttermilk, made from skim milk	□ 1 cup
evaporated low-fat milk, undiluted	□ ½ cup
nonfat dry milk, undiluted	□ ¼ cup
skim milk	□ 1 cup
yogurt, plain (made with nonfat milk)	□ 1 cup

MODERATELY LOW-FAT

buttermilk, made from whole milk	□ 1 cup
low-fat milk, 1%	□ 1 cup
yogurt, plain (made with low-fat milk)	□ 1 cup

Note: Buttermilk can be a significant source of sodium. Limit your intake of this or select no-salt-added buttermilk. If you are unable to locate it, check with your grocery store manager.

FATS

Fats are classified as either polyunsaturated, monounsaturated or saturated. Although fats are technically mixtures of these three types, they are categorized by the predominating fat in the mixture.

Remember, it is advisable to restrict your intake of total fat to less than 30 percent of your total calories for the day (see Governing Guidelines) with less than 10 percent from polyunsaturated fats, less than 10 percent from saturated fats and the balance from monounsaturated fats.

This means the ratio of one type of fat to the other should be 1:1:1. Labels found on many food items refer to a Polyunsaturated/Saturated or "P/S" ratio. You will also find the P/S ratio as part of the nutrition information in the recipe section of this book.

A P/S ratio tells you which type of fat is predominant in the food. A P/S ratio of 1 means the fats are present in balanced amounts. A P/S ratio greater than 1 means polyunsaturated fats are predominant; a P/S ratio of less than 1 means saturated fats are predominant. Choices include:

Polyunsaturated

margarine, tub, regular or unsalted (made with polyunsaturated oil)	□ 1 teaspoon
oils, vegetable (except coconut, olive, palm, palm-kernel and peanut)	□ 1 teaspoon
nuts (except Brazil, cashews, macadamia and pistachio)	□ 5
mayonnaise	□ 2 teaspoons
*salad dressings, except those containing cheese	□ 2 teaspoons
seeds: pumpkin, sunflower	□ 1 tablespoon

*Note: May be high in sodium. Check label.

Monounsaturated

margarine, liquid or stick, regular or unsalted (made with polyunsaturated oil)	□ 1 teaspoon
oils: olive, peanut	□ 1 teaspoon
olives (high in sodium)	□ 5 small
avocados	□ ⅛ small
canola or rapeseed oil	□ 1 teaspoon

SUGARS

honey	□ 2½ teaspoons
jam	□ 1 tablespoon
jelly	□ 1 tablespoon
maple syrup	□ 1 tablespoon
molasses	□ 1 tablespoon
sugar	□ 1 tablespoon

FREE FOODS

aromatic bitters
coffee
herbs and spices, with no added salt or sodium
seltzer or mineral water
tea

COUNTING CALORIES

Not only do different people have different personalities, they also have different caloric needs. These calorie requirements are based on body size, height, age, sex and activity level. To determine your personal caloric requirements to achieve or maintain ideal weight, refer to the following guidelines.

1.□ Calculate your basal caloric requirements (the energy you expend at rest) by multiplying your personal weight goal or your ideal weight (see Table IIIC) by one of the following factors:

Age	Women	Men
under 45	10	11
over 45	9	10

2.□ Adjust caloric requirements for age by subtracting 10 calories for each year over 25 from your basal energy requirement.
3.□ Add calories for physical activity by multiplying the figure derived in guideline 2 by one of the following:

□ sedentary (office work) = .3
□ moderately sedentary (occasional participation in an exercise program) = .4
□ moderately active (participation in a regular exercise program) = .5
□ extremely active (Olympic hopeful) = 1

For example, using the formula above and Table IIIC, a woman with the following characteristics—47 years of age, small frame, 5 feet 4 inches tall and sedentary—would calculate her caloric requirements as indicated below:

1.□ 140 pounds x 9 calories/pound = 1260 calories
2.□ 47 years − 25 years = 22 years
    22 years × 10 calories/year = 220 calories
    1260 calories − 220 calories = 1040 calories
3.□ 1040 calories × .3 = 312 calories
    1040 + 312 = 1352 total calories

As you can see, the less active you are, the fewer calories you can afford to eat without gaining weight.

To help you either achieve or maintain your ideal weight in a HEART SMART manner, we provide suggested diet plans for 1600 and 2000 calories that are low in fat and high in complex carbohydrates. Both diets use the HEART SMART Plan food groups for guidance in choosing the proper kinds and amounts of foods.

1.□ Refer to the food-group units that correspond to the calorie level closest to your own requirements.
2.□ Calculate your food-group units on a ratio basis.

For example, a person who requires 1850 calories would follow these steps:

a.□ Refer to the food-group units that correspond to 2000 calories.
b.□ Multiply all food-group units by 1850/2000 or 0.9250 (4 fruit-group units × 0.9250 = 3¾ fruit-group units).
c.□ It may be impractical to reduce servings by ¼ of a food-group unit, so it would be necessary to calculate as instructed, then adjust food-group units as practical.

TABLE IIIC
Height and Weight Table

		Men					Women		
Height		Small	Medium	Large	Height		Small	Medium	Large
Feet	Inches	Frame	Frame	Frame	Feet	Inches	Frame	Frame	Frame
5	2	128–134	131–141	138–150	4	10	102–111	109–121	118–131
5	3	130–136	133–143	140–153	4	11	103–113	111–123	120–134
5	4	132–138	135–145	142–156	5	0	104–115	113–126	122–137
5	5	134–140	137–148	144–160	5	1	106–118	115–129	125–140
5	6	136–142	139–151	146–164	5	2	108–121	118–132	128–143
5	7	138–145	142–154	149–168	5	3	111–124	121–135	131–147
5	8	140–148	145–157	152–172	5	4	114–127	124–138	134–151
5	9	142–151	148–160	155–176	5	5	117–130	127–141	137–155
5	10	144–154	151–163	158–180	5	6	120–133	130–144	140–159
5	11	146–157	154–166	161–184	5	7	123–136	133–147	143–163
6	0	149–160	157–170	164–188	5	8	126–139	136–150	146–167
6	1	152–164	160–174	168–192	5	9	129–142	139–153	149–170
6	2	155–168	164–178	172–197	5	10	132–145	142–156	152–173
6	3	158–172	167–182	176–202	5	11	135–148	145–159	155–176
6	4	162–176	171–187	181–207	6	0	138–151	148–162	158–179

Weights, at ages 25–29 based on lowest mortality, given in pounds according to frame (in indoor clothing weighing 5 pounds for men and 3 pounds for women; shoes with 1″-heels).

SOURCE: Metropolitan Life Insurance Company, Health and Safety Division, 1983.

For example, for 1850 calories, you may want to keep 4 fruit-group units, but will choose to reduce vegetable-group units to 4, even though when figured on a ratio basis, you would be allowed 4½ vegetables.

GOVERNING GUIDELINES

In order to increase your chances of success in reducing your risk for developing coronary heart disease, follow these tips:

1.□ Consult your physician.

2.□ Monitor your eating and activity behaviors by using the information in chapter II.

3.□ Familiarize yourself with foods that contain small or large amounts of cholesterol, fats and sodium. (See Appendices A, B, C and D.)

4.□ Follow the suggested food-group units for a diet of 1600 or 2000 calories, or calculate your own individual energy needs.

5.□ Study the sample menus that follow to assist you in designing your own diet.

MENU MAGIC

The following menus show how you can use the HEART SMART Plan food groups and diets to plan tasty, satisfying meals for the day. For your convenience, we've given you two weekday menus and one weekend menu suitable for entertaining. Your guests will appreciate your concern for their health too.

You will see that the total servings of food groups each day do not exactly match the diets for 1600 and 2000 calories provided below. The menus have been designed this way to show you that it is not necessary to follow the plans *exactly*. What is important is that you generally eat as suggested, paying more attention to the types of food you eat and the way the foods are prepared than to exact amounts. Of course, this does not mean you should eat more than suggested if you are trying to lose weight or if you find you are gaining undesired weight. Use your common sense in these matters.

FOOD GROUP	1600 CALORIES	2000 CALORIES
Vegetables	4 units	5 units
Fruit	4 units	4 units
Grains	6 units	8 units
Legumes	½ unit	1 unit
Meat and Alternatives*		
Very Low-Fat	—	1 unit
Moderately Low-Fat	3 units	3 units
Milk Products*		
Very Low-Fat	2 units	1 unit
Moderately Low-Fat	—	1 unit
Fats		
Polyunsaturated	4 units	5 units
Monounsaturated	4 units	5 units
Sugars	2 units	2 units

*Note: If the higher-fat categories are designated, it is acceptable to choose foods from the lower-fat categories. However, it is not appropriate to choose more food-group units than suggested from the higher-fat categories, unless that choice is adjusted for by choosing lower-fat categories in other groups. (See example on sample Menu Day 1, 1600 calories, where very low-fat meats are chosen and 1 moderately low-fat milk is chosen.)

THE HEART SMART
1600 CALORIE FOOD PLAN SAMPLE
WEEKDAY MENU 1

Recipes for the asterisked (*) items are found in Chapter V.

BREAKFAST

FOOD GROUPS		FOR 2000 CALORIES CHANGE AMOUNTS AS FOLLOWS:
2 Fruits	⅔ cup chilled apple juice mixed with	
Free Food	Sparkling mineral water and served over ice	
2 Grains	1 small toasted sesame-seed bagel spread with	
2 Fats, Mono-unsaturated	2 teaspoons margarine and	
1 Sugar	1 tablespoon raspberry preserves	
Free Food	Hot coffee or tea	

LUNCH

2 Vegetables	1 serving Pasta and	
1 Grain	Vegetable Salad*	
1 Fat, Mono-unsaturated		
1 Grain	1 small crusty roll, warmed	2 medium crusty rolls, warmed (Adds 1 Grain)
1 Fruit	1 serving Berry Frost*	
1 Milk Product, Very Low-Fat		
½ Sugar		

DINNER

½ Legume	1 serving Bean Dip* with	2 servings Bean Dip* (Adds ½ Legume)
1 Vegetable	½ cup fresh carrot sticks	1 cup fresh carrot sticks (Adds 1 Vegetable)
1 Vegetable 1 Grain 1 Fat, Polyun- saturated 3½ Meat and Alternatives, Very Low-Fat	1 serving Mexican Baked Fish*	
1 Grain	½ cup fluffy brown rice with	1 cup fluffy brown rice (Adds 1 Grain)
1 Vegetable 1 Fat, Mono- unsaturated	onions sautéed in 1 teaspoon olive oil	
½ Sugar	1 serving Mocha Me- ringues*	

SNACK

1 Fruit	1 chilled fresh pear, sliced and topped with	
1 Milk Prod- uct, Moder- ately Low- Fat	1 cup low-fat plain yo- gurt sprinkled with	
1 Fat, Polyun- saturated	1 tablespoon sunflower seeds	2 tablespoons sun- flower seeds (Adds 1 Fat, Poly- unsaturated)

TOTAL SERVINGS OF FOOD GROUPS FOR DAY 1:

1600 CALORIE MENU:
5 Vegetables
4 Fruits
6 Grains
½ Legume
3½ Meat and Alternatives,
   Very Low-Fat
2 Milk Products,
   1 Very Low-Fat
   1 Moderately Low-Fat
6 Fats,
   2 Polyunsaturated
   4 Monounsaturated
2 Sugars

2000 CALORIE MENU:
6 Vegetables
4 Fruits
8 Grains
1 Legume
3½ Meat and Alternatives,
   Very Low-Fat
2 Milk Products,
   1 Very Low-Fat
   1 Moderately Low-Fat
7 Fats,
   3 Polyunsaturated
   4 Monounsaturated
2 Sugars

THE HEART SMART
1600 CALORIE FOOD PLAN SAMPLE
WEEKDAY MENU 2

Recipes for the asterisked (*) items are found in Chapter V.

BREAKFAST

FOOD GROUPS		FOR 2000 CALORIES CHANGE AMOUNTS AS FOLLOWS:
1½ Grains 1 Fat, Polyun- saturated ½ Sugar	1 oven-warmed Honey Bran Muffin*	2 Honey Bran Muf- fins* (Adds 1½ Grains, 1 Fat, Polyunsat- urated, ½ Sugar)
2 Fats, Mono- unsaturated	spread with 1 teaspoon margarine	2 teaspoons marga- rine (Adds 1 Fat, Mono- unsaturated)
½ Sugar	1½ teaspoons orange marmalade	
1 Milk Prod- uct, Very Low-Fat	1 cup ice-cold skim milk	
1 Fruit	½ cup melon in season with lime slice	

LUNCH

2 Vegetables 1 Legume 1 Fat, Polyun- saturated	1 serving Split Pea Soup*	
1 Meat and Al- ternatives, Very Low-Fat	Deviled Chicken in En- dive*	
1½ Grains	4 low-fat, low-sodium whole-grain crackers	6 crackers (adds ½ Grain)
3 Fruits	1 cup unsweetened pineapple juice	

DINNER

2 Vegetables 3 Meat and Alternatives, Very Low-Fat	1 serving Veal and Peppers*	
1 Vegetable 1 Grain ½ Fat, Monounsaturated	1 serving Rice and Pasta Medley*	
1 Grain ½ Fat, Polyunsaturated	1 slice Cracked Wheat Bread*	2 slices Cracked Wheat Bread* (Adds 1 Grain, ½ Fat, Polyunsaturated)
1 Fat, Monounsaturated	1 teaspoon margarine	2 teaspoons margarine (Adds 1 Fat, Monounsaturated)

SNACK

1 Milk Product, Very Low-Fat	1 cup skim milk flavored with
Free Food	¼ teaspoon vanilla extract and
½ Sugar	1 teaspoon sugar
1 Grain	2 squares graham crackers

TOTAL SERVINGS OF FOOD GROUPS FOR DAY 2:

1600 CALORIE MENU:
5 Vegetables
4 Fruits
6 Grains
1 Legume
4 Meat and Alternatives,
   Very Low-Fat
2 Milk Products,
   Very Low-Fat
6 Fats,
   2½ Polyunsaturated
   3½ Monounsaturated
1½ Sugars

2000 CALORIE MENU:
5 Vegetables
4 Fruits
9 Grains
1 Legume
4 Meat and Alternatives,
   1 Very Low-Fat
   3 Moderately Low-Fat
2 Milk Products,
   Very Low-Fat
9½ Fats,
   4 Polyunsaturated
   5½ Monounsaturated
2 Sugars

THE HEART SMART
1600 CALORIE FOOD SAMPLE
WEEKEND MENU

Recipes for the asterisked (*) items are found in Chapter V.

BRUNCH

FOOD GROUPS		FOR 2000 CALORIES CHANGE AMOUNTS AS FOLLOWS:
1 Fruit	½ pink grapefruit with mint sprig	
1 Fruit	1 serving Whole-	2 Servings Whole-
1½ Grains	Wheat Pancakes	Wheat Pancakes
1 Fat, Polyun-	with Rosy Apple-	with Rosy Apple-
saturated	sauce* with	sauce*
		(Adds 1 Fruit, 1½ Grains, 1 Fat, Polyunsaturated)
1 Sugar	1 tablespoon maple syrup and	2 tablespoons maple syrup (Adds 1 Sugar)
2 Fats, Mono-	2 teaspoons margarine	4 teaspoons marga-
unsaturated		rine (Adds 2 Fats, Monounsaturated)
1 Milk Prod-	1 cup ice-cold skim	
uct,	milk	
Very Low-Fat		
Free Food	Hot coffee or tea	

MIDAFTERNOON SNACK

½ Vegetable	½ serving Three-Bean
¾ Legume	Bake*
2 Grains	6 small bread sticks

DINNER

1 Vegetable	1 serving Egg Drop Soup*
2 Vegetables	Chicken and Vegetable Stir Fry*
3 Meat and Alternatives, Moderately Low-Fat	
2 Vegetables	Sautéed Broccoli*
1 Fat, Monounsaturated	
2 Fruits	1 cup chilled fresh melon in season
1½ Grains	1¼ cup brown rice

EVENING SNACK

1 Fruit	1 serving Curried Fruit and Nuts*
2 Fats, Polyunsaturated	
1 Milk Product, Very Low-Fat	1 serving Irish Coffee Milk Shake*
1 Sugar	

TOTAL SERVINGS OF FOOD GROUPS FOR WEEKEND:

1600 CALORIE MENU:
5½ Vegetables
5 Fruits
5 Grains
¾ Legume
3 Meat and Alternatives, Moderately Low-Fat
2 Milk Products, Very Low-Fat
6 Fats,
  3 Polyunsaturated
  3 Monounsaturated
2 Sugars

2000 CALORIE MENU:
5½ Vegetables
6 Fruits
6½ Grains
1 Legume
4 Meat and Alternatives,
  1 Very Low-Fat
  3 Moderately Low-Fat
2 Milk Products, Very Low-Fat
9 Fats,
  4 Polyunsaturated
  5 Monounsaturated
3 Sugars

CHAPTER IV

□

FROM READING LABELS TO SETTING TABLES

□ In preceding chapters, you learned how to change your eating and exercise habits to improve your heart health. This chapter takes you further with tips on choosing and preparing foods. Specifically, it covers:

□ How to modify recipes
□ How to prepare HEART SMART foods
□ How to shop for food
□ How to choose foods in a variety of social situations

MODIFYING RECIPES FOR HEART HEALTH

Try these easy-to-follow techniques and tips for modifying and preparing your own family favorites. By using the suggested substitutions, you can significantly lower the cholesterol, fat and sodium content of standard recipes.

FOR	HEART SMART ALTERNATIVE
□ sour cream	□ low-fat yogurt
□ creamed cottage cheese (4% fat)	□ low-fat cottage cheese (1% fat), pot cheese, farmer's cheese
□ ricotta cheese	□ part-skim ricotta cheese
□ heavy cream	□ evaporated skim or low-fat milk
□ whole milk	□ low-fat milk (1–2% fat), skim milk
□ butter	□ margarine made with liquid vegetable oil
□ oil	□ olive, canola, corn, safflower, soybean, sunflower, peanut
□ salad dressings	□ nonfat or low-fat yogurt mixed with mustard, lemon, herbs and spices or oil-free dressings
□ luncheon meats	□ turkey and chicken breast
□ tuna packed in oil	□ low-sodium, water-packed tuna or water-packed, rinsed and drained
□ red meat protein sources	□ dried peas and beans (legumes), pasta, grains, cereals
□ potato chips, corn chips	□ salt-free pretzels, air-popped popcorn, rice cakes
□ chocolate candies	□ dried fruits, nuts (except Brazil, cashews, macadamia and pistachio), sesame and sunflower seeds
□ ice cream, ice milk	□ sherbet, Italian ices
□ commercial gravies	□ homemade gravies, skimmed of fat
□ self-basting turkey	□ regular turkey, basted
□ prime or choice grades of meat	□ good or standard grades of meat

FOR	HEART SMART ALTERNATIVE
□ hard cheese: Cheddar	□ low-fat cheddar or Swiss; part-skim Swiss, muenster, mozzarella; no salt added
□ chocolate cake	□ angel food cake
□ pastries	□ graham crackers, vanilla wafers
□ 1 cup solid shortening	□ ⅔ cup polyunsaturated or monounsaturated vegetable oil
□ 1 egg	□ 2 egg whites
□ cooking vegetables in butter	□ steam vegetables; flavor with herbs
□ biscuits, muffins, croissants	□ hard rolls, pita pockets, Italian bread, sandwich bread
□ high-fat crackers	□ bread sticks, graham crackers, whole-grain crackers or flat breads, melba toast, oyster crackers, soda crackers
□ sautéing foods in fat	□ sauté in nonstick skillet without oil or use skillet sprayed with nonstick cooking spray
□ browning meats in fat	□ brown in its own fat
□ preparing gravies	□ chill until fat congeals and lift off fat, or dip paper towel in gravy to absorb fat, or use a gravy skimmer
□ cooking poultry	□ remove skin, then cook as recipe directs
□ cooking meats	□ trim all visible fat from meat prior to cooking; cook on a rack to drain fat
□ buttering breads, muffins and vegetables	□ dip a pastry brush in olive or sesame oil and lightly paint breads, muffins and vegetables

FOR	HEART SMART ALTERNATIVE
□ poaching meat, fish and poultry in cream sauce	□ use vegetable stock or clear, low-sodium broth
□ purchasing beef	□ choose lean cuts: loin, chuck, ground beef, flank steak
□ purchasing pork	□ choose lean cuts: pork pieces, arm roast, loin
□ purchasing lamb	□ choose lean cuts: leg, loin, rib, shoulder
□ purchasing veal	□ choose lean cuts: cutlets, sirloin roast, veal breast
□ purchasing fish	□ choose varieties high in omega-3 fatty acids at least 2 times per week (See Appendix D)

SUPERMARKET SURVIVAL

It's often said that healthful eating takes too much time in planning and shopping and costs too much for the average budget. But don't believe it. Healthful eating can be accomplished easily and within a budget by following many of the guidelines below.

□ Plan menus; then make a list to enable you to recall all necessary HEART SMART grocery items. Recipe preparation goes much faster when you have all necessary ingredients on hand.

□ Eat before you shop to avoid impulse buying of non-HEART SMART foods.

□ Use coupons and comparison shop to save money.

□ Buy store brands or no frills to economize on HEART SMART foods.

□ Larger sizes are usually, but not always, the best buy.

□ Read labels to become familiar with the products you buy and eat. The information on labels can help you take advantage of specials by telling you whether the food will fit into your diet.

In reading the ingredient list on food labels, you may come across a number of words that are unfamiliar. Some of these "foreign" words should become familiar to you. For example, although a number of ingredients do not contain the word "fat" in their names, they are in fact high in fat content, particularly saturated fat. Such ingredient names include:

□ glycerol
□ hydrogenated shortening
□ lard
□ coconut and coconut oil
□ palm oil and palm-kernel oil

These notorious fats are often found in breads and crackers. A label may read "Prepared with 100% vegetable oil," yet contain coconut, palm or palm-kernel oils which are saturated fats. Nondairy creamers and whipped toppings also contain coconut oil.

Any ingredients that contain the word "sodium" should also be noted. The more mention there is of sodium, the more likely the food should be avoided. Examples of sodium compounds include sodium chloride (salt), monosodium glutamate, sodium bicarbonate (baking soda), baking powder, disodium phosphate, sodium alginate, sodium benzoate, sodium hydroxide, sodium nitrite, sodium propianate and sodium sulfite.

Many of these sodium compounds are used as preservatives in food items and should be limited in your diet. The order in which ingredients appear is important. Listed by weight, an ingredient that appears at the beginning of the list is the ingredient in greatest quantity. Canned products usually contain high amounts of sodium. Purchase fresh or frozen or the low-salt variety. Be aware of hidden sodium found in common medications such as antacids and some prescription medications. Ask your doctor or dietitian for advice about a particular food or medication if you are uncertain. If your doctor has prescribed potassium supplements for you, be aware that many salt substitutes and low-sodium products contain potassium chloride in place of sodium. Consult your doctor or dietitian about your recommended potassium intake.

Now that you will be making heart-healthier food choices, the supermarket shelves are brimming with possibilities.

There are a number of new oils that may be of interest to you for their exotic tastes. Examples are walnut oil, almond oil, sesame oil and canola or rapeseed oil. Bear in mind that food companies have responded to the consumer's need for healthier, lower fat, cholesterol and sodium products. You can find low-sodium versions of such condiments as soy sauce and Worcestershire, and cheeses with reduced fat or salt. These products are sometimes found in dietetic and specialty sections of your grocery store, or they may be found alongside traditional versions.

SOCIAL SITUATION SAVVY

Do you feel your busy schedule doesn't allow you to follow HEART SMART guidelines? Do you seem to have less control over your food choices at social occasions? Help is on the way. It *is* possible to diet in all social situations. But remember, no one can do it for you; you must do it for yourself. Make these promises to yourself to enhance your social-situation savvy:

□ Be aggressive. Do not allow people to talk you into eating foods you know you shouldn't have.

□ Eat a light meal or snack before attending a special function where food is plentiful. By fasting before such a gathering, you tend to eat too much.

□ Do not feel obligated to join the "clean plate club." Rid yourself of food guilt; you will be doing yourself a favor by helping to make your heart healthy.

RESTAURANT REMEDIES

□ When at least one of your daily meals is eaten away from home, you may wonder how you can "stick to" your heart-healthy menu plan. The good news is that many restaurants, even fast food restaurants and airline food service, offer a wide array of choices.

□ If possible, contact the restaurant in advance. Ask about the foods available, and ask if special requests will be honored. Many restaurants will prepare dishes with margarine instead of butter; trim fats from meats; and broil, bake, steam or poach entrees. Airlines usually have dietetic meals available. Simply call and reserve yours.

□ Read menus carefully and question the waiter or waitress if you have any concerns about a method of cooking or ingredient. Here are some tips on reading menus:

—Look for words that indicate low-fat preparation: "steamed," "garden fresh," "broiled," "roasted," "poached," "in its own juice."

—Be wary of high sodium terms: "pickled," "smoked," "cocktail sauce," "cured," or "in broth."

—Avoid: "buttery," "buttered," "in butter sauce," "fried," "sautéed," "panfried," "crispy,"

"creamed," "in cream," "hollandaise," "au gratin,"
"escalloped," "Parmesan."
□ Choose an appetizer such as seafood cocktail, raw
vegetables or fresh fruit. Avoid salty tomato juice and
soups.
□ If you wish to have a cocktail, remember that alcohol
adds empty calories. Order your drink with water,
juice or low-calorie soda rather than presweetened
mixes. Choose a wine spritzer or, better yet,
sparkling water with a twist of lime.
□ Choose raw or steamed vegetables and salads to
increase your fiber and complex carbohydrate intake.
Avoid creamy dressings, bacon, croutons and egg
toppings on salads.
□ If you cannot possibly turn down a favorite dessert,
eat only half.

ETHNIC IS IN

□ Ethnic restaurants are in. Chinese restaurants
provide many good choices. Avoid egg foo yung, fried
egg noodles, salty soups and oily Szechuan foods.
Instead, try boiled, steamed or stir-fried dishes with
soy sauce on the side. Order without MSG
(monosodium glutamate). Enjoy lots of rice.
□ Indian cuisine is well suited to the HEART SMART
Plan. Many dishes use a yogurt-based curry sauce,
and a variety of low-fat salads are available. Lentils
and other low-fat beans such as chick-peas are Indian
staples and make good choices.
□ Italian restaurants offer fare that is suitable for your
diet. Choose marsala sauce instead of cream, and try
simply prepared chicken or fish dishes. Order pasta
with a small amount of margarine or olive oil. Order
Italian ices for dessert.

□ Mexican can be a boost for your diet. Avoid high-fat fried tortillas, and start out with tomato, onion and avocado salad or plain rice and beans (not refried). They're great sources of fiber. Order a tamale (steamed, not fried) filled with chicken or beans. Many restaurants offer steamed or broiled fish or fish stews. Be sure to order condiments like sour cream and cheese on the side.

□ In fast food restaurants, look for simply prepared items: salad bars (beware of the croutons, bacon and dressings, though), fresh fruit. If you *must* have a burger, choose the regular (2-ounce) hamburger with lettuce, tomato and onion but without mayonnaise or catsup. Avoid the fried foods, double-decker burgers and pickles.

These are just examples of the many ways you can sample restaurant fare and keep your HEART SMART Plan on track. Balance, variety and moderation are the keys to healthier living. Do it today, and you will be helping to make your heart healthier for today and tomorrow.

In an ideal world, television commercials would urge Americans to eat nutritious diets, not junk diets. Vending machines would contain fruit juices and nutritious snacks, rather than sugary soft drinks and fatty candy bars. Labels on all processed foods would boldly state fat, sugar and salt content. Restaurants specializing in low-cholesterol cuisine would become fashionable all over the country.

As you know, it's a far from perfect world. But you're learning to change part of it to suit yourself and the needs of your increasingly healthy body.

CHAPTER V

□

RECIPES FOR A MORE HEALTHY HEART

□ The HEART SMART recipes do more than show you how to put the plan into action. They're tasty and sure to satisfy the whole family. With them, it is easy to plan a diet, not only for the person in your household who has been diagnosed as needing cholesterol reduction, but also for the rest of the family. Try them and enjoy good eating for your heart's health!

APPETIZERS

DEVILED CHICKEN IN ENDIVE

¾ cup (5 ounces) chopped,
  cooked chicken
2 tablespoons plain low-fat
  yogurt
1 tablespoon finely chopped
  green onion
1 teaspoon mayonnaise

1 teaspoon dry mustard
  powder
⅛ teaspoon salt
⅛ teaspoon ground black
  pepper
8 Belgian endive leaves
Chopped parsley for garnish
  (optional)

□ In small bowl, combine chicken, yogurt, green onion, mayonnaise, mustard, salt and pepper. Cover and refrigerate about 1 hour. Before serving, spoon an equal amount of mixture on wide end of each endive leaf. Sprinkle with chopped parsley (if desired). **MAKES 8 SERVINGS.**

APPROXIMATE NUTRIENT ANALYSIS PER SERVING:

Calories □ 40
Protein □ 6 grams
Fat □ 1 gram
Carbohydrate □ 1 gram
Cholesterol □ 15 milligrams
Sodium □ 25 milligrams
Potassium □ 135 milligrams

% Calories from Fat □ 28
% Calories from Saturated Fat
  □ 8
% Calories from
  Monounsaturated Fat □ 9
% Calories from Polyunsaturated
  Fat □ 11
P/S □ 1.4

FOOD GROUP UNITS:

Meat and Alternatives:
  Very Low-Fat □ 1

CURRIED FRUIT AND NUTS

⅓ cup (about 40) whole
blanched almonds
½ cup (about 24) walnut
halves
¾ cup raisins, plumped in
water

2 tablespoons margarine
1 teaspoon curry powder
⅛ teaspoon ground red
pepper

□ Preheat oven to 325°F. In medium-size bowl, combine almonds, walnuts and drained raisins.

In small saucepan over low heat, melt margarine. Add curry and red pepper and cook, stirring frequently, 1 minute. Pour over nut mixture; toss well.

Spray baking pan with nonstick cooking spray. Spread mixture on pan. Bake 15 to 20 minutes or until nuts are lightly browned, stirring occasionally. Spread on wax paper to cool. May be served warm or at room temperature. **MAKES 8 SERVINGS**, about ¼ cup each.

APPROXIMATE NUTRIENT ANALYSIS PER SERVING:

Calories □ 145
Protein □ 3 grams
Fat □ 10 grams
Carbohydrate □ 13 grams
Cholesterol □ 0
Sodium □ 40 milligrams
Potassium □ 185 milligrams

% Calories from Fat □ 59
% Calories from Saturated Fat
□ 7
% Calories from
Monounsaturated Fat □ 24
% Calories from Polyunsaturated
Fat □ 28
P/S □ 3.8

FOOD GROUP UNITS:

Fruits □ 1

Fat:
Polyunsaturated □ 2

EGGPLANT CAVIAR

2 tablespoons olive oil
2 cups chopped eggplant (¾-
    1 pound, untrimmed)
¼ cup finely chopped onion
2 garlic cloves, minced
2 medium tomatoes, peeled,
    chopped (1 cup)
1½ tablespoons fresh lemon
    juice

½ teaspoon dried oregano
½ teaspoon ground cumin
⅛ teaspoon salt
⅛ teaspoon ground black
    pepper
Unsalted whole-grain crackers

□ In large nonstick skillet over high heat, heat olive oil. Add eggplant, onion and garlic and cook, stirring occasionally, 5 minutes or until soft. Add remaining ingredients, except crackers; cover. Cook, stirring occasionally, 20 to 25 minutes. Transfer to small bowl; cover. Refrigerate about 1 hour. Serve with crackers. **MAKES 8 SERVINGS**, about ¼ cup each.

APPROXIMATE NUTRIENT ANALYSIS PER SERVING:

Calories □ 55
Protein □ 1 gram
Fat □ 4 grams
Carbohydrate □ 5 grams
Cholesterol □ 0
Sodium □ 35 milligrams
Potassium □ 195 milligrams

% Calories from Fat □ 57
% Calories from Saturated Fat
    □ 8
% Calories from
    Monounsaturated Fat □ 43
% Calories from Polyunsaturated
    Fat □ 6
P/S □ 0.7

FOOD GROUP UNITS:

Vegetables □ 1

Fat:
    Monounsaturated □ ½

STUFFED CHERRY TOMATOES

16 cherry tomatoes (½ pint container)
1 can (3¼ ounces) low-sodium tuna in water, drained and flaked (¾ cup)
2 tablespoons plain low-fat yogurt
2 teaspoons finely chopped green onion
2 teaspoons low-sodium chili sauce
¼ teaspoon prepared horseradish
⅛ teaspoon ground black pepper

□ With a sharp knife, slice tops of tomatoes. With a grapefruit spoon, remove pulp; drain upside down on paper towels.

In small bowl, combine remaining ingredients. Spoon an equal amount into each tomato. Refrigerate about 1 hour. MAKES 4 SERVINGS.

APPROXIMATE NUTRIENT ANALYSIS PER SERVING:

Calories □ 60
Protein □ 8 grams
Fat □ 1 gram
Carbohydrate □ 7 grams
Cholesterol □ 9 milligrams
Sodium □ 30 milligrams
Potassium □ 360 milligrams

% Calories from Fat □ 11
% Calories from Saturated Fat □ 3
% Calories from Monounsaturated Fat □ 2
% Calories from Polyunsaturated Fat □ 6
P/S □ 2.5

FOOD GROUP UNITS:

Vegetables □ ½
Meat and Alternatives:
  Very Low-Fat □ ½

MEXICAN CHEESE DIP

1 cup plain low-fat yogurt
½ cup low-fat cottage cheese
2 tablespoons unsalted
  margarine
1 garlic clove, minced

2 tablespoons chopped green
  chilies
1 teaspoon chili powder
⅛ teaspoon ground black
  pepper

□ In small bowl, combine all ingredients. Cover and refrigerate about 1 hour. Stir well before serving. Serve with assorted fresh vegetables. **MAKES 6 SERVINGS**, about ½ cup each.

APPROXIMATE NUTRIENT ANALYSIS PER SERVING:

Calories □ 75
Protein □ 4 grams
Fat □ 5 grams
Carbohydrate □ 4 grams
Cholesterol □ 3 milligrams
Sodium □ 110 milligrams
Potassium □ 120 milligrams

% Calories from Fat □ 56
% Calories from Saturated Fat
  □ 16
% Calories from
  Monounsaturated Fat □ 24
% Calories from Polyunsaturated
  Fat □ 16
P/S □ 1.0

FOOD GROUP UNITS:

Meat and Alternatives:
  Moderately Low-Fat □ ½

Fat:
  Polyunsaturated □ ½

Mushroom Pâté

2 tablespoons unsalted
  margarine
¼ cup finely chopped onion
  (½ small)
¼ cup finely chopped green
  pepper
1 garlic clove, minced
½ cup low-fat cottage cheese
2 eggs

1 pound mushrooms, finely
  chopped
¾ cup plain, dry, salt-free
  bread crumbs
½ teaspoon dried basil
½ teaspoon dried oregano
¼ teaspoon dried thyme
⅛ teaspoon ground black
  pepper

□ Preheat oven to 325°F. Spray pan with nonstick cooking spray. In small skillet over medium-high heat, melt margarine. Add onion, green pepper and garlic and cook, stirring frequently, about 4 minutes or until soft; set aside.

In large bowl with mixer at medium speed, beat cottage cheese and eggs until smooth. Stir in remaining ingredients and onion mixture until well combined. Spoon into pan. Bake 1½ to 2 hours or until firm to touch. Cool on wire rack 30 minutes. Remove from pan. Cover and refrigerate overnight. MAKES 10 SERVINGS.

APPROXIMATE NUTRIENT ANALYSIS PER SERVING:

Calories □ 90
Protein □ 5 grams
Fat □ 4 grams
Carbohydrate □ 9 grams
Cholesterol □ 55 milligrams
Sodium □ 65 milligrams
Potassium □ 225 milligrams

% Calories from Fat □ 41
% Calories from Saturated Fat
  □ 10
% Calories from
  Monounsaturated Fat □ 19
% Calories from Polyunsaturated
  Fat □ 12
P/S □ 1.1

FOOD GROUP UNITS:

Vegetables □ 1
Grains □ ½

Fat:
  Polyunsaturated □ 1

PITA CRISPS

2 small whole-wheat pita
   pocket breads
1 tablespoon + 1 teaspoon
   margarine, melted
½ teaspoon dried oregano

⅛ teaspoon dried thyme
⅛ teaspoon garlic powder
1 teaspoon poppy seeds

□ Preheat oven to 400°F. Split each pita bread in half. Cut each half into 8 triangles.

In small bowl, combine margarine, oregano, thyme and garlic powder; brush evenly over each pita triangle; place on baking sheet. Sprinkle with poppy seeds. Bake about 10 to 15 minutes or until crisp. **MAKES 4 SERVINGS.**

APPROXIMATE NUTRIENT ANALYSIS PER SERVING:

Calories □ 170
Protein □ 6 grams
Fat □ 5 grams
Carbohydrate □ 28 grams
Cholesterol □ 0
Sodium □ 125 milligrams
Potassium □ 175 milligrams

% Calories from Fat □ 25
% Calories from Saturated Fat
   □ 5
% Calories from
   Monounsaturated Fat □ 9
% Calories from Polyunsaturated
   Fat □ 11
P/S □ 2.5

FOOD GROUP UNITS:

Grains □ 1

Fat:
   Polyunsaturated □ 1

BEAN DIP

1 cup cooked (about ½ cup
  dried) or canned, drained
  and rinsed kidney beans
2 tablespoons minced onion
1 garlic clove , minced
1 tablespoon plain low-fat
  yogurt
1 teaspoon mayonnaise

2 tablespoons chopped green
  pepper
⅛ teaspoon dry mustard
  powder
1 teaspoon sugar
2 teaspoons tomato paste
⅛ teaspoon salt

□ In blender or food processor at medium speed, purée all ingredients until smooth; place in small bowl. Cover and refrigerate about 2 hours. Let stand at room temperature about 20 minutes before serving. MAKES 8 SERVINGS, about 2 tablespoons each.

APPROXIMATE NUTRIENT ANALYSIS PER SERVING:

Calories □ 40
Protein □ 2 grams
Fat □ 1 gram
Carbohydrate □ 7 grams
Cholesterol □ 0
Sodium □ 40 milligrams
Potassium □ 115 milligrams

% Calories from Fat □ 13
% Calories from Saturated Fat
  □ 3
% Calories from
  Monounsaturated Fat □ 4
% Calories from Polyunsaturated
  Fat □ 6
P/S □ 2.8

FOOD GROUP UNITS:

Legumes □ ½

HUMMUS

1 cup dried chick-peas
1 quart water
1 bay leaf
2 tablespoons chopped fresh
   parsley
1 tablespoon + 1 teaspoon
   sesame tahini
1 tablespoon fresh lemon
   juice

1 tablespoon olive oil
2 garlic cloves, chopped
¼ teaspoon salt
Additional chopped fresh
   parsley for garnish
   (optional)
Pita bread or raw vegetables

□ Place chick-peas in 2-quart saucepan with water to cover. Soak overnight. Drain; return to saucepan. Add 1 quart water and bay leaf. Bring to a boil. Reduce heat, cover and simmer until tender, about 1½ hours. Drain, reserving about ¼ cup liquid. Place chick-peas and 3 tablespoons reserved liquid in food processor with remaining ingredients, except garnish. Process until smooth, scraping sides of bowl with spatula if necessary. If mixture is too thick, add additional tablespoon cooking liquid. Garnish with parsley (if desired). Serve with pita bread or raw vegetables. **MAKES 10 SERVINGS**, about ¼ cup each.

APPROXIMATE NUTRIENT ANALYSIS PER SERVING:

Calories □ 100
Protein □ 5 grams
Fat □ 4 grams
Carbohydrate □ 13 grams
Cholesterol □ 0
Sodium □ 55 milligrams
Potassium □ 185 milligrams

% Calories from Fat □ 32
% Calories from Saturated Fat
   □ 5
% Calories from
   Monounsaturated Fat □ 17
% Calories from Polyunsaturated
   Fat □ 10
P/S □ 1.9

FOOD GROUP UNITS:

Legumes □ ½
Meat and Alternatives:
   Very Low-Fat □ ½

Fat:
   Monounsaturated □ ½

GUACAMOLE

1¼ pound avocado, peeled, cut into chunks (about 2½ cups)
1 large tomato (6 ounces), peeled, seeded, cut into eighths
½ cup chopped green pepper
½ cup chopped onion
½ cup plain low-fat yogurt
1 tablespoon fresh lemon juice
½ teaspoon chili powder
⅛ teaspoon salt

□ Place all ingredients in food processor and process until blended, scraping sides of bowl if necessary. Chill before serving. MAKES 14 SERVINGS, about ¼ cup each.

APPROXIMATE NUTRIENT ANALYSIS PER SERVING:

Calories □ 85
Protein □ 2 grams
Fat □ 7 grams
Carbohydrate □ 5 grams
Cholesterol □ 1 milligram
Sodium □ 30 milligrams
Potassium □ 320 milligrams

% Calories from Fat □ 72
% Calories from Saturated Fat □ 13
% Calories from Monounsaturated Fat □ 50
% Calories from Polyunsaturated Fat □ 9
P/S □ 0.7

FOOD GROUP UNITS:

Vegetables □ 1

Fat:
Monounsaturated □ 1½

BEVERAGES

TOMATO SIZZLER

½ cup low-sodium vegetable
  juice cocktail
½ cup crushed ice
½ teaspoon prepared
  horseradish

⅛ teaspoon hot-pepper sauce
⅛ teaspoon celery seed
1 celery rib

□ In blender at low speed, blend all ingredients about 30 seconds. Pour into glass. Garnish with celery rib. **MAKES 1 SERVING.**

APPROXIMATE NUTRIENT ANALYSIS PER SERVING:

Calories □ 30
Protein □ 0
Fat □ 0
Carbohydrate □ 0
Cholesterol □ 0
Sodium □ 60 milligrams
Potassium □ 295 milligrams

% Calories from Fat □ 0

FOOD GROUP UNITS:

Vegetables □ 1

CARROT-PINEAPPLE JUICE

¾ cup shredded carrots (1
  large)
½ cup water

1 can (8 ounces) crushed
  pineapple in juice
½ cup crushed ice

□ In blender at medium speed, blend carrots and water about 1 minute. Strain; return liquid to blender. Add remaining ingredients; blend at low speed until smooth. Pour into two glasses. **MAKES 2 SERVINGS.**

APPROXIMATE NUTRIENT ANALYSIS PER SERVING:

Calories □ 85
Protein □ 2 grams
Fat □ 0
Carbohydrate □ 45 grams
Cholesterol □ 0
Sodium □ 30 milligrams
Potassium □ 545 milligrams

% Calories from Fat □ 0

FOOD GROUP UNITS:

Fruits □ 2

BERRY FROST

¾ cup frozen unsweetened
   strawberries, slightly thawed
½ cup plain low-fat yogurt
¼ cup skim milk

1 teaspoon sugar
1 teaspoon vanilla extract
1 ice cube

□ In blender at low speed, blend all ingredients until smooth and frothy; pour into glass. **MAKES 1 SERVING.**

APPROXIMATE NUTRIENT ANALYSIS PER SERVING:

Calories □ 150
Protein □ 9 grams
Fat □ 2 grams
Carbohydrate □ 23 grams
Cholesterol □ 8 milligrams
Sodium □ 115 milligrams
Potassium □ 550 milligrams

% Calories from Fat □ 14
% Calories from Saturated Fat
   □ 8
% Calories from
   Monounsaturated Fat □ 4
% Calories from Polyunsaturated
   Fat □ 2
P/S □ 0.2

FOOD GROUP UNITS:

Fruits □ 1

Sugars □ ½

COCO-BANANA SHAKE

½ cup skim milk
½ cup plain low-fat yogurt
½ small ripe banana, mashed
1 teaspoon sugar

½ teaspoon vanilla extract
¼ teaspoon coconut extract
1 ice cube

□ In blender at low speed, blend all ingredients about 30 seconds; pour into glass. MAKES 1 SERVING.

APPROXIMATE NUTRIENT ANALYSIS PER SERVING:

Calories □ 190
Protein □ 11 grams
Fat □ 2 grams
Carbohydrate □ 32 grams
Cholesterol □ 9 milligrams
Sodium □ 145 milligrams
Potassium □ 705 milligrams

% Calories from Fat □ 11
% Calories from Saturated Fat
  □ 7
% Calories from
  Monounsaturated Fat □ 3
% Calories from Polyunsaturated
  Fat □ 1
P/S □ 0.1

FOOD GROUP UNITS:

Fruits □ 1
Milk Products:
  Moderately Low-Fat □ 1

RICH MOCHA COCOA

1 cup skim milk
1 cinnamon stick
2 teaspoons unsweetened
  cocoa powder

2 teaspoons sugar
1 teaspoon instant coffee
  powder
¼ teaspoon vanilla extract

□ In small saucepan over low heat, cook milk and cinnamon stick about 5 minutes. In small bowl, combine cocoa, sugar and coffee powder. With whisk, blend mixture into milk; add vanilla. Cook, stirring frequently, about 2 minutes. Remove and discard cinnamon stick; pour into mug. MAKES 1 SERVING.

APPROXIMATE NUTRIENT ANALYSIS PER SERVING:

Calories □ 135
Protein □ 9 grams
Fat □ 1 gram
Carbohydrate □ 24 grams
Cholesterol □ 4 milligrams
Sodium □ 130 milligrams
Potassium □ 535 milligrams

% Calories from Fat □ 6
% Calories from Saturated Fat
 □ 3
% Calories from
 Monounsaturated Fat □ 2
% Calories from Polyunsaturated
 Fat □ 1
P/S □ 0.1

FOOD GROUP UNITS:

Grains □ ½
Milk Products:
 Very Low-Fat □ 1

RASPBERRY FRAPPE

1½ cups orange juice
½ cup fresh raspberries
1 teaspoon sugar

1 egg white
1 cup crushed ice

□ In blender at high speed, blend orange juice, raspberries, sugar and egg white about 30 seconds. Gradually add ice, blending until thick and frothy; pour into glasses. **MAKES 4 SERVINGS.**

APPROXIMATE NUTRIENT ANALYSIS PER SERVING:

Calories □ 55
Protein □ 2 grams
Fat □ 0
Carbohydrate □ 13 grams
Cholesterol □ 0
Sodium □ 15 milligrams
Potassium □ 220 milligrams

% Calories from Fat □ 0

FOOD GROUP UNITS:

Fruits □ 1

IRISH COFFEE MILKSHAKE

½ cup skim milk
½ cup plain low-fat yogurt
2 teaspoons sugar

1 teaspoon instant coffee
  powder
1 teaspoon Irish whiskey

□ In blender at low speed, blend all ingredients about 30 seconds. Pour into glass. MAKES 1 SERVING.

APPROXIMATE NUTRIENT ANALYSIS PER SERVING:

Calories □ 160
Protein □ 10 grams
Fat □ 2 grams
Carbohydrate □ 23 grams
Cholesterol □ 9 milligrams
Sodium □ 145 milligrams
Potassium □ 565 milligrams

% Calories from Fat □ 11
% Calories from Saturated Fat
  □ 7
% Calories from
  Monounsaturated Fat □ 3
% Calories from Polyunsaturated
  Fat □ 1
P/S □ 0

FOOD GROUP UNITS:

Milk Products:
  Very Low-Fat □ 1

Sugars □ 1

SPICED ICED TEA

3 cups cold water
4 tea bags
1½ tablespoons sugar
1 cinnamon stick, broken into
  pieces

2 whole cloves
1 orange slice
Ice cubes

□ In medium-size saucepan, heat water to boiling. Remove from heat; add remaining ingredients. Cover and let steep 5 to 7 minutes. Strain and pour tea into tall glasses filled with ice cubes. MAKES 4 SERVINGS, about ⅔ cup each.

APPROXIMATE NUTRIENT ANALYSIS PER SERVING:

Calories □ 15   % Calories from Fat □ 0
Protein □ 0
Fat □ 0
Carbohydrate □ 5 grams
Cholesterol □ 0
Sodium □ 1 milligram
Potassium □ 50 milligrams

FOOD GROUP UNITS:

Sugars □ ½

SOUPS

CREAM OF POTATO SOUP

2 tablespoons unsalted
  margarine
½ cup chopped onion
¼ cup chopped celery
1½ cups peeled diced
  potatoes (1 large)
1 cup low-sodium chicken
  broth

¼ cup chopped fresh parsley
¼ teaspoon dried thyme
¼ teaspoon celery seed
⅛ teaspoon ground black
  pepper
1½ cups skim milk

□ In medium-size saucepan over medium-high heat, melt margarine. Add onion and celery and cook, stirring frequently, 4 minutes or until soft. Add potatoes, chicken broth, parsley, thyme, celery seed and pepper; bring to a boil. Reduce heat, cover and simmer 15 minutes or until potatoes are almost tender. Add milk; simmer uncovered, stirring occasionally, 5 minutes.

In blender at medium speed, blend about a quarter of the mixture at a time until smooth. Return to saucepan; heat about 1 minute. MAKES 4 SERVINGS, about 1 cup each.

APPROXIMATE NUTRIENT ANALYSIS PER SERVING:

Calories □ 130
Protein □ 7 grams
Fat □ 6 grams
Carbohydrate □ 14 grams
Cholesterol □ 2 milligrams
Sodium □ 90 milligrams
Potassium □ 345 milligrams

% Calories from Fat □ 41
% Calories from Saturated Fat
   □ 9
% Calories from
   Monounsaturated Fat □ 18
% Calories from Polyunsaturated
   Fat □ 14
P/S □ 1.6

FOOD GROUP UNITS:

Grains □ 1
Milk Products:
   Very Low-Fat □ ½

Fat:
   Polyunsaturated □ 1

CORN CHOWDER

2 tablespoons unsalted
   margarine
¼ cup chopped onion
¼ cup chopped red pepper
1 tablespoon all-purpose flour

2 cups skim milk
1⅓ cups frozen whole-kernel
   corn
¼ teaspoon dried thyme
⅛ teaspoon ground black
   pepper

□ In medium-size saucepan over medium-high heat, melt margarine. Add onion and red pepper and cook, stirring frequently, 4 minutes or until soft. Add flour; cook, stirring constantly, about 1 minute. Gradually add milk, corn, thyme and pepper. Reduce heat to low; cook 5 to 7 minutes or until slightly thickened and corn is tender. MAKES 4 SERVINGS, about ⅔ cup each.

APPROXIMATE NUTRIENT ANALYSIS PER SERVING:

Calories □ 150
Protein □ 6 grams
Fat □ 6 grams
Carbohydrate □ 20 grams
Cholesterol □ 2 milligrams
Sodium □ 65 milligrams
Potassium □ 320 milligrams

% Calories from Fat □ 34
% Calories from Saturated Fat
   □ 7
% Calories from
   Monounsaturated Fat □ 16
% Calories from Polyunsaturated
   Fat □ 10
P/S □ 1.5

VEGETABLE SOUP

1 tablespoon vegetable oil
½ cup chopped onion
2 garlic cloves, minced
1 can (16 ounces) tomatoes,
  canned without salt,
  chopped
1 cup low-sodium chicken
  broth
1 cup sliced carrots (about 2
  medium)

1 cup sliced celery
¼ cup chopped fresh parsley
1 teaspoon dried basil
⅛ teaspoon pepper
1 cup frozen, no-salt-added
  lima beans
½ cup water

□ In medium-size saucepan over medium-high heat, heat oil. Add onion and garlic and cook, stirring frequently, 2 to 3 minutes or until soft. Add tomatoes with their juice, chicken broth, carrots, celery, parsley, basil and pepper; bring to a boil. Reduce heat, cover and simmer 20 minutes. Add lima beans and water; bring to a boil. Reduce heat; simmer 20 minutes or until beans are tender. MAKES 6 SERVINGS, about ¾ cup each.

APPROXIMATE NUTRIENT ANALYSIS PER SERVING:

Calories □ 90
Protein □ 5 grams
Fat □ 3 grams
Carbohydrate □ 14 grams
Cholesterol □ 0
Sodium □ 60 milligrams
Potassium □ 460 milligrams

% Calories from Fat □ 26
% Calories from Saturated Fat
  □ 4
% Calories from
  Monounsaturated Fat □ 6.5
% Calories from Polyunsaturated
  Fat □ 15.5
P/S □ 4.2

FOOD GROUP UNITS:

Vegetables □ 2
Legumes □ ¼

Fat:
 Polyunsaturated □ ½

ONION SOUP

2 tablespoons unsalted
 margarine
2 cups thinly sliced onion (2
 medium)
1 tablespoon all-purpose flour

4 cups low-sodium beef broth
⅛ teaspoon ground black
 pepper
4 tablespoons freshly grated
 Parmesan cheese

□ In large saucepan over low heat, melt margarine. Add onion and cook, stirring frequently, 15 minutes. Add flour and cook, stirring constantly, 1 minute. Add broth and pepper; bring to a boil.

Reduce heat, cover and simmer, stirring occasionally, 25 minutes or until onions are very soft. Sprinkle with Parmesan cheese. **MAKES 4 SERVINGS, about 1 cup each.**

APPROXIMATE NUTRIENT ANALYSIS PER SERVING:

Calories □ 130
Protein □ 5 grams
Fat □ 8 grams
Carbohydrate □ 10 grams
Cholesterol □ 5 milligrams
Sodium □ 125 milligrams
Potassium □ 745 milligrams

% Calories from Fat □ 54
% Calories from Saturated Fat
 □ 16
% Calories from
 Monounsaturated Fat □ 23
% Calories from Polyunsaturated
 Fat □ 15
P/S □ 0.8

FOOD GROUP UNITS:

Vegetables □ 2

Fat:
 Polyunsaturated □ 1½

GAZPACHO

1 cup fresh whole-wheat
  bread crumbs (2 slices)
2 tablespoons red wine
  vinegar
2 tablespoons vegetable oil
2 garlic cloves, minced
1 cup seeded, diced
  cucumber

½ cup diced green pepper
2 tablespoons finely chopped
  green onion
3 cups peeled, seeded,
  chopped tomatoes (5-6)
1 cup tomato juice
⅛ teaspoon ground black
  pepper

□ In small bowl, combine bread crumbs, vinegar, oil and garlic; mix to a smooth paste.

In large bowl, combine remaining ingredients; stir in bread paste until well blended. Cover and refrigerate about 4 hours. **MAKES 6 SERVINGS**, about ⅔ cup each.

APPROXIMATE NUTRIENT ANALYSIS PER SERVING:

Calories □ 100
Protein □ 3 grams
Fat □ 5 grams
Carbohydrate □ 13 grams
Cholesterol □ 0
Sodium □ 70 milligrams
Potassium □ 455 milligrams

% Calories from Fat □ 43
% Calories from Saturated Fat
  □ 6
% Calories from
  Monounsaturated Fat □ 11
% Calories from Polyunsaturated
  Fat □ 26
P/S □ 4.3

FOOD GROUP UNITS:

Vegetables □ 1
Grains □ ½

Fat:
  Polyunsaturated □ 1

DILLED CARROT BISQUE

2 cups low-sodium chicken
  broth
2 cups sliced carrots (3
  medium carrots)
¼ cup chopped fresh parsley
2 tablespoons chopped
  shallots

1 garlic clove, minced
½ teaspoon dried dill weed
⅛ teaspoon ground black
  pepper
½ cup skim milk

□ In medium-size saucepan over medium-high heat, combine chicken broth, carrots, parsley, shallots, garlic, dill weed and pepper; bring to a boil. Reduce heat, cover and simmer 30 minutes or until carrots are tender.

In blender or food processor at medium speed, blend about a quarter of the mixture at a time until smooth. Return to saucepan; stir in milk and heat about 1 minute. Do not boil. MAKES 3 SERVINGS, about ¾ cup each.

APPROXIMATE NUTRIENT ANALYSIS PER SERVING:

Calories □ 75
Protein □ 9 grams
Fat □ 1 gram
Carbohydrate □ 12 grams
Cholesterol □ 1 milligram
Sodium □ 130 milligrams
Potassium □ 360 milligrams

% Calories from Fat □ 12
% Calories from Saturated Fat
  □ 5
% Calories from
  Monounsaturated Fat □ 3
% Calories from Polyunsaturated
  Fat □ 4
P/S □ 0.9

FOOD GROUP UNITS:

Vegetables □ 2
Milk Products: Very Low-Fat □ ¼

SPLIT PEA SOUP

2 tablespoons unsalted
  margarine
1 cup chopped carrots
½ cup chopped onion
2 garlic cloves, minced
4½ cups water
1½ cups dry split peas

1 bay leaf
1 tablespoon dry white wine
1 teaspoon white vinegar
½ teaspoon salt
½ teaspoon dried thyme
⅛ teaspoon ground black
  pepper

☐ In large saucepan over medium-high heat, melt margarine. Add carrots, onion, garlic and cook, stirring frequently, 4 minutes or until soft. Add remaining ingredients; bring to a boil. Reduce heat, cover and simmer, stirring occasionally, 1 to 1¼ hours. If soup becomes too thick, add additional water. Remove and discard bay leaf. **MAKES 6 SERVINGS**, about ¾ cup each.

APPROXIMATE NUTRIENT ANALYSIS PER SERVING:

Calories ☐ 195
Protein ☐ 11 grams
Fat ☐ 5 grams
Carbohydrate ☐ 30 grams
Cholesterol ☐ 0
Sodium ☐ 175 milligrams
Potassium ☐ 475 milligrams

% Calories from Fat ☐ 20
% Calories from Saturated Fat
  ☐ 4
% Calories from
  Monounsaturated Fat ☐ 9
% Calories from Polyunsaturated
  Fat ☐ 7
P/S ☐ 1.7

FOOD GROUP UNITS:

Vegetables ☐ 2
Legumes ☐ 1

Fat:
  Polyunsaturated ☐ 1

FISH CHOWDER

1 tablespoon olive oil
½ cup chopped onion
½ cup chopped green pepper
½ cup sliced celery
1 large garlic clove, minced
1 can (16 ounces) tomatoes,
  canned without salt
1–1½ cups water
⅓ cup sherry
1 cup peeled, diced potatoes
  (6 ounces)

½ cup sliced carrots
¼ cup chopped fresh parsley
1 bay leaf
1 teaspoon dried basil
½ teaspoon dried thyme
⅛–¼ teaspoon ground black
  pepper
⅛ teaspoon salt
12 ounces fresh or frozen,
  slightly thawed halibut, cut
  into bite-size pieces

□ In 2- or 3-quart saucepan over medium-high heat, heat oil. Add onion, green pepper, celery and garlic, and cook, stirring, 1 minute. Add tomatoes, 1 cup water, wine, potatoes, carrots, parsley, bay leaf, basil, thyme, pepper and salt. Bring to a boil. Reduce heat, cover and simmer 20 to 25 minutes or until vegetables are tender. If soup is too thick, add additional ½ cup water. Add halibut and continue cooking, covered, 10 minutes, until fish is opaque. Remove bay leaf before serving. MAKES 6 SERVINGS, about 1 cup each.

APPROXIMATE NUTRIENT ANALYSIS PER SERVING:

Calories □ 115
Protein □ 11 grams
Fat □ 4 grams
Carbohydrate □ 12 grams
Cholesterol □ 14 milligrams
Sodium □ 90 milligrams
Potassium □ 585 milligrams

% Calories from Fat □ 26
% Calories from Saturated Fat
  □ 4
% Calories from
  Monounsaturated Fat □ 16
% Calories from Polyunsaturated
  Fat □ 6
P/S □ 1.2

FOOD GROUP UNITS:

Vegetables □ 1
Grains □ ⅓
Meat and Alternatives:
  Very Low-Fat □ 1½

Fat:
  Monounsaturated □ ½

MUSHROOM-BARLEY SOUP

2 tablespoons canola oil
1 large onion, chopped (1
  cup)
2 garlic cloves, minced
1 medium parsnip, peeled (4
  ounces)
1½ cups sliced carrots (3
  medium)
12 ounces sliced fresh
  mushrooms
6 cups water
½ cup uncooked barley

⅓ cup sherry cooking wine
4 packets low-sodium beef
  broth and seasoning mix
1½ tablespoons low-sodium
  soy sauce
1 bay leaf
¼–½ teaspoon ground black
  pepper
¼ teaspoon dried thyme
¼ cup chopped fresh parsley

□ In 3- or 4-quart saucepan over medium-high heat, heat oil. Add onion and garlic and cook, stirring, 1 minute. Add parsnip and carrots and cook, stirring, 1 minute. Add mushrooms and cook, stirring, 2 to 3 minutes or until tender. Add water, barley, wine, broth and seasoning mix, soy sauce, bay leaf, pepper, thyme and salt. Stir to blend. Bring to a boil. Reduce heat, cover and simmer 50 to 55 minutes or until barley is tender. Remove bay leaf. Garnish with parsley. MAKES 8 SERVINGS, about 1 cup each.

APPROXIMATE NUTRIENT ANALYSIS PER SERVING:

Calories □ 125
Protein □ 3 grams
Fat □ 4 grams

% Calories from Fat □ 27
% Calories from Saturated Fat
  □ 3

Carbohydrate □ 21 grams
Cholesterol □ 0
Sodium □ 125 milligrams
Potassium □ 670 milligrams

% Calories from
  Monounsaturated Fat □ 16
% Calories from Polyunsaturated
  Fat □ 8
P/S □ 3.5

FOOD GROUP UNITS:

Grains □ 1
Vegetables □ 1

Fat:
  Monounsaturated □ 1

EGG DROP SOUP

4 cups low-sodium chicken
  broth, divided
1 cup shredded Chinese
  cabbage
2 tablespoons chopped green
  onion
¼ teaspoon ground ginger

Dash pepper
1 tablespoon cornstarch
1 egg white
1 tablespoon water

□ In medium-size saucepan, combine 3¾ cups chicken broth, cabbage, green onion, ginger and pepper; bring to a boil.

In small bowl, combine remaining chicken broth and cornstarch until well blended. Add to saucepan and cook, stirring occasionally, about 5 minutes. Beat egg white and water. Pour egg into saucepan slowly, stirring slightly with a fork to form threads. Cook about 1 minute. MAKES 4 SERVINGS, about 1 cup each.

APPROXIMATE NUTRIENT ANALYSIS PER SERVING:

Calories □ 45
Protein □ 11 grams
Fat □ 6 grams

% Calories from Fat □ 19
% Calories from Saturated Fat
  □ 5.5

Carbohydrate □ 18 grams
Cholesterol □ 0
Sodium □ 135 milligrams
Potassium □ 250 milligrams

% Calories from
  Monounsaturated Fat □ 3
% Calories from Polyunsaturated
  Fat □ 10.5
P/S □ 1.6

FOOD GROUP UNITS:

Vegetables □ 1
Meat and Alternatives:
  Very Low-Fat □ ¼

MAIN DISHES

VEGETABLE PIZZA

1½ cups whole-wheat flour,
  divided
1 teaspoon active dry yeast
1 teaspoon sugar
½ cup warm water (120-
  130°F)
1 tablespoon olive oil, divided
½ pound mushrooms, sliced
  (about 2¾ cups)

⅓ cup chopped onion
1 can (8 ounces) low-sodium
  tomato sauce
1 small green pepper, cut into
  rings
4 ounces shredded part-skim
  mozzarella cheese
1 tablespoon freshly grated
  Parmesan cheese

□ In medium-size bowl, combine ¾ cup flour, yeast and sugar; add water and 2 teaspoons oil. With mixer at low speed, beat until flour is just moistened. Gradually stir in remaining flour to make a soft dough.

On lightly floured surface, knead dough 5 minutes or until smooth and elastic. Place dough in greased bowl, turning to expose greased portion. Cover with towel; set aside in warm place to rise 45 minutes or until doubled.

Meanwhile, in large nonstick skillet over medium-high heat, heat remaining oil. Add mushrooms and onion and cook, stirring occasionally, 5 minutes or until tender.

Punch down dough. Spray 12-inch round pizza pan with nonstick cooking spray. Form dough to fit pan. Spread tomato sauce over dough. Arrange green pepper rings. Sprinkle with mushroom-onion mixture. Sprinkle with mozzarella and Parmesan cheeses. Bake 15 to 20 minutes or until crust is browned. MAKES 8 SERVINGS.

APPROXIMATE NUTRIENT ANALYSIS PER SERVING:

Calories □ 155
Protein □ 8 grams
Fat □ 5 grams
Carbohydrate □ 22 grams
Cholesterol □ 9 milligrams
Sodium □ 90 milligrams
Potassium □ 235 milligrams

% Calories from Fat □ 26
% Calories from Saturated Fat
□ 11.5
% Calories from
Monounsaturated Fat □ 11.5
% Calories from Polyunsaturated
Fat □ 3
P/S □ 0.2

FOOD GROUP UNITS:

Vegetables □ 1
Grains □ 1
Meat and Alternatives:
Moderately Low-Fat □ ½

Fat:
Monounsaturated □ ½

Pasta & Bean Stew

1 tablespoon olive oil
2 large garlic cloves, minced
2 cups fresh mushrooms,
   halved
1 cup sliced carrots
2¼ cups water
⅓ cup sherry cooking wine
2 packets low-sodium beef-
   flavored broth and
   seasoning mix
1 cup uncooked small pasta
   shells
¼ cup minced fresh parsley
1 teaspoon dried basil

1 teaspoon grated lemon peel
¾ teaspoon dried tarragon
½ teaspoon dried oregano
⅛ teaspoon ground black
   pepper
Dash red pepper flakes
½ package (8 ounces) frozen
   small onions (about 1¾
   cups)
1¼ cups cooked (½ cup
   dried) or canned, rinsed
   and drained chick-peas
1¼ cups frozen sweet green
   peas
2 tablespoons freshly grated
   Parmesan cheese (optional)

□ In medium-size saucepan over medium-high heat, heat oil. Add garlic and cook, stirring, 30 seconds. Add mushrooms and carrots and cook, stirring, about 3 minutes or until mushrooms begin to soften. Add water, wine and broth and seasoning mix; bring to a boil. Stir in pasta, parsley and seasonings. Reduce heat, cover and simmer 10 minutes. Add onions, chick-peas and green peas. Simmer, covered, 10 to 15 minutes or until vegetables are tender. Sprinkle with Parmesan cheese (if desired). MAKES 6 SERVINGS, about 1 cup each.

APPROXIMATE NUTRIENT ANALYSIS PER SERVING:

Calories □ 215
Protein □ 10 grams
Fat □ 4 grams
Carbohydrate □ 36 grams
Cholesterol □ 2 milligrams
Sodium □ 90 milligrams
Potassium □ 665 milligrams

% Calories from Fat □ 18
% Calories from Saturated Fat
   □ 5
% Calories from
   Monounsaturated Fat □ 10
% Calories from Polyunsaturated
   Fat □ 3
P/S □ 0.4

RICE AND PASTA MEDLEY

1 tablespoon margarine
½ cup chopped onion
½ cup chopped celery
½ cup brown rice
2 ounces vermicelli, broken up (¾ cup)
1¼ cups low-sodium chicken broth

½ cup water
¼ cup dry white wine
¼ teaspoon salt
½ teaspoon dried thyme
⅛ teaspoon ground black pepper
¼ cup chopped fresh parsley

□ In large nonstick skillet over medium-high heat, melt margarine. Add onion and celery and cook, stirring occasionally, 3 minutes or until soft. Add rice and vermicelli and cook, stirring occasionally, until lightly browned. Add remaining ingredients, except parsley; bring to a boil. Reduce heat, cover and simmer 30 to 40 minutes or until rice is tender. Stir in parsley. MAKES 6 SERVINGS, about ½ cup each.

STUFFED PEPPERS

1 tablespoon vegetable oil
¾ cup chopped onion
½ cup chopped carrots
½ cup chopped celery
1 garlic clove, minced
2¼ cups low-sodium beef
  broth
½ teaspoon dried oregano
¼ teaspoon dried basil

⅛ teaspoon ground black
  pepper
1 cup uncooked barley
6 green peppers (about 2¼
  pounds)
½ cup low-sodium tomato
  sauce
1½ ounces shredded part-
  skim mozzarella cheese (¼
  cup + 2 tablespoons)

□ In medium-size saucepan over medium-high heat, heat oil. Add onion, carrots, celery and garlic and cook, stirring occasionally, about 5 minutes. Add beef broth, oregano, basil and pepper; bring to a boil. Add barley; reduce heat. Cover; simmer, stirring occasionally, 1 hour or until barley is tender.

Meanwhile, remove tops and seeds from peppers. In large saucepan in 1 inch boiling water, heat peppers to boiling. Reduce heat to low; cover. Simmer 5 to 7 minutes or until tender-crisp.

Preheat oven to 375°F. Arrange peppers in 1½-quart shallow baking dish. Stir tomato sauce into barley mixture. Spoon an equal amount of filling into each pepper, approximately ¾ cup. Sprinkle with cheese. Cover and bake 20 to 25 minutes. MAKES 6 SERVINGS.

APPROXIMATE NUTRIENT ANALYSIS PER SERVING:

Calories □ 225
Protein □ 8 grams
Fat □ 4 grams
Carbohydrate □ 42 grams
Cholesterol □ 4 milligrams
Sodium □ 80 milligrams
Potassium □ 795 milligrams

% Calories from Fat □ 16
% Calories from Saturated Fat
  □ 5
% Calories from
  Monounsaturated Fat □ 4
% Calories from Polyunsaturated
  Fat □ 7
P/S □ 1.3

FOOD GROUP UNITS:

Vegetables □ 2½
Grains □ 2
Meat and Alternatives:
  Moderately Low-Fat □ ½

Fat:
  Polyunsaturated □ ½

ORIENTAL-STYLE LENTIL BURGERS

1 cup dried lentils
1 cup fresh whole-wheat
  bread crumbs (2 slices)
¾ cup finely grated carrots (3
  medium)
½ cup minced scallions (4
  medium)
¼ cup finely chopped canned
  water chestnuts (about ⅓ of
  an 8-ounce can, drained)
¼ cup finely chopped celery
2 garlic cloves, minced
2 tablespoons whole-wheat
  flour

1 tablespoon low-sodium soy
  sauce
1 large egg, slightly beaten
½ teaspoon grated fresh
  ginger (or ¼ teaspoon
  ground ginger)
2–3 teaspoons canola oil
4 whole-wheat pita pocket
  breads, halved
Special Sauce (recipe follows)
2 ounces alfalfa sprouts

□ Place lentils in large pot with water to cover; let stand 1 hour. Cook lentils and water, covered, about 40 to 45 minutes or until tender. Meanwhile, prepare the remaining ingredients for burgers and Special Sauce.

Drain lentils well. There will be about 3 cups. In large bowl, combine lentils, bread crumbs, carrots, scallions, water chestnuts, celery, garlic, flour, soy sauce, egg and ginger until well blended. Refrigerate 1 hour.

Combine ingredients for Special Sauce (see below).

To cook burgers: Measure ½ cup mixture for each burger and gently shape into a 4-inch patty; mixture will be moist. Over medium-high heat, heat a large skillet. Brush with oil. Add patties and cook 3 to 4 minutes. Using 2 spatulas, turn gently. Cook 2 minutes. Reduce heat to low and cook, covered, 2 to 3 minutes or until heated through.

To serve: Place each patty in pita pocket bread half, top with alfalfa sprouts and about 1 tablespoon Special Sauce. MAKES 8 SERVINGS.

SPECIAL SAUCE

½ cup plain low-fat yogurt
½–¾ teaspoon dry mustard
2 teaspoons honey

□ Combine ingredients in small bowl; stir to blend well. Refrigerate. MAKES 8 SERVINGS, about 1 tablespoon each.

APPROXIMATE NUTRIENT ANALYSIS PER SERVING:

Calories □ 290
Protein □ 15 grams
Fat □ 4 grams
Carbohydrate □ 52 grams
Cholesterol □ 35 milligrams
Sodium □ 225 milligrams
Potassium □ 510 milligrams

% Calories from Fat □ 12
% Calories from Saturated Fat
□ 3
% Calories from
Monounsaturated Fat □ 4
% Calories from Polyunsaturated
Fat □ 5
P/S □ 1.8

FOOD GROUP UNITS:

Grains □ 2
Vegetables □ 2
Legumes □ 1
Meat and Alternatives:
Very Low-Fat □ ½

Fat:
Monounsaturated □ ½

TUNA PASTA BAKE

2 teaspoons vegetable oil
½ cup chopped onion
1 garlic clove, minced
1 can (8 ounces) low-sodium
   tomato sauce
½ teaspoon dried oregano
4 ounces spaghetti (2 cups
   cooked)

1 can (7 ounces) low-sodium
   tuna in water, drained and
   flaked
½ cup cooked peas
1 cup low-fat cottage cheese
1 egg, slightly beaten
¼ teaspoon pepper
1½ tablespoons wheat germ

□ In small saucepan over medium-high heat, heat oil. Add onion and garlic and cook, stirring occasionally, about 3 minutes. Add tomato sauce and oregano; bring to a boil. Reduce heat, cover and simmer, stirring occasionally, about 15 minutes.

Meanwhile, cook spaghetti according to package directions but without salt. Drain; place in medium bowl. Add tuna and peas; toss well.

Preheat oven to 375°F. Spray 1½-quart baking dish with nonstick cooking spray. In small bowl, combine cottage cheese, egg and pepper. Pour over spaghetti; mix well. Place mixture in baking dish. Pour sauce over mixture. Sprinkle with wheat germ. Bake 30 minutes or until hot and bubbly. **MAKES 4 SERVINGS.**

APPROXIMATE NUTRIENT ANALYSIS PER SERVING:

Calories □ 295
Protein □ 29 grams
Fat □ 6 grams
Carbohydrate □ 32 grams
Cholesterol □ 88 milligrams
Sodium □ 300 milligrams
Potassium □ 345 milligrams

% Calories from Fat □ 19
% Calories from Saturated Fat
  □ 5
% Calories from
  Monounsaturated Fat □ 6
% Calories from Polyunsaturated
  Fat □ 8
P/S □ 1.8

FOOD GROUP UNITS:

Vegetables □ 2

Grains □ 1½

Meat and Alternatives:
  Very Low-Fat □ 3

Fat:
  Polyunsaturated □ ½

THREE-BEAN BAKE

1 tablespoon canola oil
1 cup chopped onion
1 cup chopped green pepper
1 large garlic clove, minced
1 can (28 ounces) tomatoes,
  canned without salt
1¼ cups cooked (½ cup
  dried) or canned, rinsed
  and drained chick-peas
1¼ cups cooked (½ cup
  dried) or canned, rinsed
  and drained white kidney
  beans or Great Northern
  beans
¾ cup cooked (about ⅓ cup
  dried) or canned, rinsed
  and drained red kidney
  beans
1 tablespoon chili powder

¼ teaspoon ground cumin
⅛ teaspoon ground black
  pepper
¾ cup cornmeal
1 tablespoon sugar
¼ teaspoon baking soda
⅓ cup skim milk
1 egg, slightly beaten
1 tablespoon unsalted
  margarine, melted

□ Spray 2-quart casserole with nonstick cooking spray. In medium-size saucepan over medium-high heat, heat oil. Add onion, green pepper and garlic and cook, stirring, about 3 minutes. Add tomatoes, chick-peas, white and red kidney beans, chili powder, cumin and pepper. Cover and simmer, stirring occasionally, 10 minutes. Pour mixture into casserole.

Preheat oven to 375°F. In small bowl, stir together

cornmeal, sugar and baking soda. Stir in milk, egg and margarine; blend well. Spoon over top of beans. Bake 20 to 25 minutes or until cornmeal mixture is lightly browned. **MAKES 8 SERVINGS.**

APPROXIMATE NUTRIENT ANALYSIS PER SERVING:

Calories □ 205
Protein □ 8 grams
Fat □ 5 grams
Carbohydrate □ 33 grams
Cholesterol □ 35 milligrams
Sodium □ 70 milligrams
Potassium □ 560 milligrams

% Calories from Fat □ 22
% Calories from Saturated Fat
　□ 4
% Calories from
　Monounsaturated Fat □ 10
% Calories from Polyunsaturated
　Fat □ 8
P/S □ 1.7

Food Group Units:

Vegetables □ 1
Legumes □ 1
Grains □ 1

Fat:
　Monounsaturated □ 1

Mexican Tortilla Casserole

1 tablespoon canola oil
1 cup chopped onion
½ cup chopped green pepper
1 large garlic clove, minced
1 can (14½ ounces) no-salt-
　added stewed tomatoes
¼ cup dry red wine
1 teaspoon chili powder
¼ teaspoon ground cumin
¼ teaspoon ground black
　pepper

6 corn tortillas
1 cup part-skim ricotta cheese
1 large egg white
1¼ cups cooked (½ cup
　dried) or canned, rinsed
　and drained kidney beans
¼ cup grated part-skim
　mozzarella cheese
1 tablespoon freshly grated
　Parmesan cheese (optional)

□ In medium-size saucepan over medium-high heat, heat oil. Add onion, green pepper and garlic, and cook, stirring, about 3 minutes. Add tomatoes, wine, chili powder, cumin and black pepper; bring to a boil. Reduce heat, cover and simmer, stirring occasionally, 20 minutes.

Preheat oven to 350°F. Spray bottom of 2-quart casserole with nonstick cooking spray. Spread a small amount of sauce in casserole. Add 3 tortillas, spreading to cover bottom. In small bowl, blend ricotta cheese and egg white until smooth. Spread half of mixture over tortillas. Add half the beans; top with half the remaining sauce. Repeat. Top with mozzarella and Parmesan (if desired). Cover and bake 40 minutes or until bubbly. MAKES 6 SERVINGS.

APPROXIMATE NUTRIENT ANALYSIS PER SERVING:

Calories □ 235
Protein □ 13 grams
Fat □ 8 grams
Carbohydrate □ 30 grams
Cholesterol □ 15 milligrams
Sodium □ 150 milligrams
Potassium □ 480 milligrams

% Calories from Fat □ 30
% Calories from Saturated Fat
   □ 11
% Calories from
   Monounsaturated Fat □ 12
% Calories from Polyunsaturated
   Fat □ 7
P/S □ 0.3

FOOD GROUP UNITS:

Grains □ 1
Vegetables □ 1
Legumes □ ½
Meat and Alternatives:
   Moderately Low-Fat □ 1

Fat:
   Monounsaturated □ ½

VEGETARIAN CHILI WITH SOYBEANS

1 cup dried soybeans (2½ cups cooked)
¾ cup dried kidney beans (2 cups cooked)
2 pounds fresh tomatoes, peeled, chopped (2 cups)
2 cups sliced carrots
1½ cups chopped onions
1 cup chopped green pepper
2 garlic cloves, minced
1 can (6 ounces) tomato paste, canned without salt
½ cup water

1 tablespoon chili powder
1 tablespoon low-sodium soy sauce
½ teaspoon ground cumin
½ teaspoon ground black pepper
½ teaspoon dried oregano
Ground red pepper to taste (optional)
4 cups brown rice
Additional chopped onion for garnish (optional)

□ In separate large saucepans, soak soybeans and kidney beans in water to cover overnight. (Or, bring to a boil, remove from heat and let stand 1 hour.) Over low heat, cook, covered, until tender. Drain kidney beans and set aside. Drain soybeans and place in 3-quart saucepan with tomatoes, carrots, onions, green pepper, garlic, tomato paste, water, chili powder, soy sauce, cumin, black pepper, oregano and ground red pepper (if desired). Bring to a boil. Reduce heat, cover and simmer, stirring occasionally, 2 to 2½ hours, until mixture is thick and flavors are well blended. Stir in kidney beans and cook 15 minutes or until heated through. Serve on brown rice with additional chopped onion (if desired). MAKES 8 SERVINGS, about 1 cup each.

APPROXIMATE NUTRIENT ANALYSIS PER SERVING:

Calories □ 320
Protein □ 16 grams
Fat □ 5 grams

% Calories from Fat □ 13
% Calories from Saturated Fat
□ 2

Carbohydrate □ 58 grams
Cholesterol □ 0
Sodium □ 125 milligrams
Potassium □ 1200 milligrams

% Calories from
  Monounsaturated Fat □ 3
% Calories from Polyunsaturated
  Fat □ 8
P/S □ 3.6

FOOD GROUP UNITS:

Legumes □ 1½
Grains □ 1
Vegetables □ 2

KASHA AND MUSHROOMS

1 tablespoon unsalted
  margarine
½ cup chopped onion
¼ cup sliced celery
¼ pound mushrooms, sliced
  (1½ cups)
½ cup kasha (buckwheat
  groats)

1 egg white, slightly beaten
1 cup low-sodium chicken
  broth
¼ teaspoon dried rosemary
⅛ teaspoon ground black
  pepper

□ In large nonstick skillet over medium-high heat, melt margarine. Add onion and celery and cook, stirring occasionally, about 4 minutes. Add mushrooms and cook, stirring frequently, about 5 minutes. Combine kasha and egg white; add to skillet and cook, stirring frequently, about 2 minutes. Add remaining ingredients; bring to a boil. Reduce heat, cover and simmer 15 to 20 minutes or until all liquid is absorbed. MAKES 4 SERVINGS.

APPROXIMATE NUTRIENT ANALYSIS PER SERVING:

Calories □ 100
Protein □ 6 grams
Fat □ 4 grams

% Calories from Fat □ 31
% Calories from Saturated Fat
  □ 6

Carbohydrate □ 13 grams
Cholesterol □ 0
Sodium □ 60 milligrams
Potassium □ 205 milligrams

% Calories from
  Monounsaturated Fat □ 14
% Calories from Polyunsaturated
  Fat □ 11
P/S □ 1.8

FOOD GROUP UNITS:

Vegetables □ ½
Grains □ 1

Fat:
  Polyunsaturated □ ½

EGGPLANT LASAGNA

1 medium eggplant, cut into
  very thin slices (1½ pounds)
1 tablespoon vegetable oil
½ cup chopped onion
1 pound mushrooms, sliced
9 lasagna noodles

1 jar (15½ ounces) no-salt-
  added spaghetti sauce
8 ounces part-skim ricotta
  cheese (1 cup)
4 ounces shredded part-skim
  mozzarella cheese (1 cup)
2 tablespoons freshly grated
  Parmesan cheese

□ Spray large nonstick skillet with nonstick cooking spray. Add eggplant slices and brown; set aside. In same skillet, heat oil. Add onion and cook, stirring occasionally, about 3 minutes. Add mushrooms and cook, stirring frequently, 5 to 7 minutes or until mushrooms are tender.

Cook lasagna noodles according to package directions but without salt.

Preheat oven to 350°F. Spoon ¼ cup sauce into 11- × 7-inch baking dish. Arrange three alternating layers of noodles, ricotta, mushroom mixture, mozzarella cheese, eggplant slices, sauce and Parmesan cheese. Cover and bake 30 to 40 minutes or until heated through. MAKES 8 SERVINGS.

APPROXIMATE NUTRIENT ANALYSIS PER SERVING:

Calories □ 290
Protein □ 15 grams
Fat □ 9 grams
Carbohydrate □ 40 grams
Cholesterol □ 19 milligrams
Sodium □ 160 milligrams
Potassium □ 490 milligrams

% Calories from Fat □ 27
% Calories from Saturated Fat
  □ 13
% Calories from
  Monounsaturated Fat □ 8
% Calories from Polyunsaturated
  Fat □ 6
P/S □ 0.4

FOOD GROUP UNITS:

Vegetables □ 2
Grains □ 2
Meat and Alternatives:
  Moderately Low-Fat □ 1½

Fat:
  Polyunsaturated □ ½

WHOLE-WHEAT PANCAKES WITH ROSY APPLESAUCE

4 small red apples, cored and
  sliced
6 tablespoons water, divided
2 tablespoons sugar
1 teaspoon fresh lemon juice
⅛ teaspoon ground cinnamon
Dash ground cloves
⅓ cup whole-wheat flour

⅓ cup all-purpose flour
1¼ teaspoons baking powder
½ cup low-fat milk
1 egg, slightly beaten
2 teaspoons vegetable oil
1½ teaspoons vanilla extract

□ In medium-size saucepan over low heat, combine apples, 3 tablespoons water, sugar, lemon juice, cinnamon and cloves; bring to a boil. Reduce heat, cover and simmer 7 to 10 minutes or until apples are tender. Push mixture through a strainer into bowl. Cover and refrigerate until ready to use.

Preheat a nonstick griddle or griddle sprayed with nonstick cooking spray. In small bowl, combine whole-wheat and all-purpose flour and baking powder. Stir in remaining ingredients and 3 tablespoons water until flour is moistened. Spoon 2 tablespoons of batter per pancake onto hot griddle; cook until golden brown on both sides. Serve with warm or chilled applesauce. MAKES 5 SERVINGS, 2 pancakes each.

APPROXIMATE NUTRIENT ANALYSIS PER SERVING:

Calories □ 185
Protein □ 4 grams
Fat □ 4 grams
Carbohydrate □ 35 grams
Cholesterol □ 56 milligrams
Sodium □ 110 milligrams
Potassium □ 220 milligrams

% Calories from Fat □ 18
% Calories from Saturated Fat
  □ 5
% Calories from
  Monounsaturated Fat □ 5
% Calories from Polyunsaturated
  Fat □ 8
P/S □ 1.6

FOOD GROUP UNITS:

Fruits □ 1
Grains □ 1½

Fat:
  Polyunsaturated □ 1

RED SNAPPER STEW

1 tablespoon vegetable oil
1 cup sliced celery (2 medium
  stalks)
1 cup sliced carrots (2
  medium)
½ cup chopped onion
½ cup chopped green pepper
2 garlic cloves, minced
1 can (16 ounces) tomatoes,
  canned without salt,
  chopped

1 cup low-sodium chicken
  broth
¼ cup dry white wine
½ teaspoon dried dill weed
1 bay leaf
¼ teaspoon ground black
  pepper
1½ pounds red snapper fillets,
  cut into 1-inch pieces
½ cup water

□ In medium-size saucepan over medium-high heat, heat oil. Add celery, carrots, onion, green pepper and garlic and cook, stirring occasionally, about 10 minutes or until tender-crisp. Add tomatoes with their juice, chicken broth, wine, dill, bay leaf and pepper; bring to a boil. Reduce heat, cover and simmer about 20 minutes. Add fish and water; bring to a boil. Reduce heat and simmer 10 minutes or until fish flakes. Remove and discard bay leaf. MAKES 6 SERVINGS, about 1 cup each.

APPROXIMATE NUTRIENT ANALYSIS PER SERVING:

Calories □ 170
Protein □ 26 grams
Fat □ 4 grams
Carbohydrate □ 9 grams
Cholesterol □ 45 milligrams
Sodium □ 135 milligrams
Potassium □ 705 milligrams

% Calories from Fat □ 22
% Calories from Saturated Fat
□ 5
% Calories from
Monounsaturated Fat □ 6
% Calories from Polyunsaturated
Fat □ 11
P/S □ 2.2

FOOD GROUP UNITS:

Vegetables □ 2
Meat and Alternatives:
Very Low-Fat □ 3

Fat:
Polyunsaturated □ ½

SOLE FLORENTINE

1 package (10 ounces) fresh or no-salt-added frozen spinach
4 sole fillets (1 pound)
1½ tablespoons unsalted margarine
2 tablespoons chopped onion
2 tablespoons all-purpose flour

1 cup skim milk
⅛ teaspoon ground black pepper
Dash ground nutmeg
1 teaspoon freshly grated Parmesan cheese
⅛ teaspoon paprika

□ Preheat oven to 350°F. Cook spinach according to package directions but without salt. Spray 8-inch square baking dish with nonstick cooking spray. Arrange spinach in baking dish. Arrange fillets in single layer over spinach.

In small saucepan over low heat, melt margarine. Add onion and cook, stirring frequently, 3 minutes or until soft. Add flour and cook, stirring frequently, about 1 minute. Gradually add milk, pepper and nutmeg and cook, stirring constantly, until thickened and smooth. Pour over fish. Sprinkle with cheese and paprika. Bake 15 minutes or until fish flakes. MAKES 4 SERVINGS.

APPROXIMATE NUTRIENT ANALYSIS PER SERVING:

Calories □ 265
Protein □ 31 grams
Fat □ 6 grams
Carbohydrate □ 9 grams
Cholesterol □ 44 milligrams
Sodium □ 300 milligrams
Potassium □ 1020 milligrams

% Calories from Fat □ 25
% Calories from Saturated
  Fat □ 7
% Calories from
  Monounsaturated Fat □ 10
% Calories from Polyunsaturated
  Fat □ 8
P/S □ 1.5

FOOD GROUP UNITS:

Vegetables □ 1
Meat and Alternatives:
  Very Low-Fat □ 3
Milk Products:
  Very Low-Fat □ ¼

Fat:
  Polyunsaturated □ ½

CRUMB-TOPPED FILLETS

2 tablespoons unsalted
  margarine, melted
2 tablespoons minced onion
1 tablespoon fresh lemon
  juice
3 walnut halves, chopped
1 small garlic clove, minced
½ teaspoon dried Italian
  seasoning

⅛ teaspoon ground black
  pepper
4 trout fillets (1 pound)
½ teaspoon paprika
¼ cup fresh whole-wheat
  bread crumbs (about 1
  slice)
Fresh parsley sprigs for garnish

☐ In small bowl, combine margarine, onion, lemon juice, walnuts, garlic, Italian seasoning and pepper; mix well. Spoon an equal amount of mixture over each fillet. Sprinkle with paprika; top with bread crumbs. Spray broiler rack with nonstick cooking spray. Place fish on rack. Broil 3 to 4 inches from heat 5 to 7 minutes or until topping is lightly browned and fish flakes easily. Garnish with parsley. **MAKES 4 SERVINGS.**

APPROXIMATE NUTRIENT ANALYSIS PER SERVING:

Calories ☐ 250
Protein ☐ 21 grams
Fat ☐ 10 grams
Carbohydrate ☐ 5 grams
Cholesterol ☐ 60 milligrams
Sodium ☐ 110 milligrams
Potassium ☐ 50 milligrams

% Calories from Fat ☐ 35
% Calories from Saturated Fat
  ☐ 7
% Calories from
  Monounsaturated Fat ☐ 14
% Calories from Polyunsaturated
  Fat ☐ 14
P/S ☐ 1.9

FOOD GROUP UNITS:

Meat and Alternatives:
  Very Low-Fat ☐ 3

Fat:
  Polyunsaturated ☐ ½

Fillets En Papillote

4 flounder fillets (1 pound)
1 cup chopped tomatoes (2 medium)
¼ cup minced green pepper
2 tablespoons minced onion
2 garlic cloves, minced

¼ teaspoon grated lemon peel
2 teaspoons fresh lemon juice
½ teaspoon dried basil
⅛ teaspoon ground black pepper
4 teaspoons unsalted margarine

□ Preheat oven to 350°F. Place each fillet on aluminum foil or parchment paper. Sprinkle each fillet with equal amounts of tomato, green pepper, onion, garlic, lemon peel, lemon juice, basil and pepper. Top each fillet with 1 teaspoon margarine. Wrap and seal all edges; place on baking pan. Bake 20 minutes or until fish flakes. MAKES 4 SERVINGS, about 3 ounces fish each.

APPROXIMATE NUTRIENT ANALYSIS PER SERVING:

Calories □ 225
Protein □ 27 grams
Fat □ 5 grams
Carbohydrate □ 5 grams
Cholesterol □ 43 milligrams
Sodium □ 210 milligrams
Potassium □ 685 milligrams

% Calories from Fat □ 26
% Calories from Saturated Fat □ 6
% Calories from Monounsaturated Fat □ 11
% Calories from Polyunsaturated Fat □ 9
P/S □ 1.7

Food Group Units:

Vegetables □ 1
Meat and Alternatives:
    Very Low-Fat □ 3

Fat:
    Polyunsaturated □ ½

COLD POACHED SALMON WITH CURRY SAUCE

½ cup dry white wine
⅓ cup water
1 bay leaf
4-5 whole peppercorns
4 salmon steaks (1 pound)

½ cup plain low-fat yogurt
2 teaspoons mayonnaise
1 tablespoon finely chopped
 green onion
¾ teaspoon curry powder
⅛ teaspoon ground cumin

□ In large skillet, combine wine, water, bay leaf and pepper; bring to a boil. Add salmon, cover and simmer, turning once, 5 to 7 minutes or until fish flakes. Transfer to platter. Cover and refrigerate about 2 hours.

In small bowl, combine remaining ingredients. Serve with salmon. **MAKES 4 SERVINGS**, about 3 ounces salmon each.

APPROXIMATE NUTRIENT ANALYSIS PER SERVING:

Calories □ 190
Protein □ 25 grams
Fat □ 9 grams
Carbohydrate □ 2 grams
Cholesterol □ 43 milligrams
Sodium □ 130 milligrams
Potassium □ 460 milligrams

% Calories from Fat □ 42
% Calories from Saturated Fat
 □ 9
% Calories from
 Monounsaturated Fat □ 20
% Calories from Polyunsaturated
 Fat □ 13
P/S □ 1.4

FOOD GROUP UNITS:

Meat and Alternatives:
 Very Low-Fat □ 3

Fat:
 Polyunsaturated □ ½

SWEET AND SOUR FILLETS

1 ½ teaspoons vegetable oil
2 tablespoons chopped onion
2 tablespoons chopped red
    pepper
1 small garlic clove, minced
¼ cup water
1 tablespoon red wine vinegar
1 tablespoon sugar

1 ½ teaspoons dry sherry
¾ teaspoon low-sodium soy
    sauce
Dash pepper
4 bass fillets, cut in half* (1
    pound)
1 teaspoon cornstarch
    dissolved in 2 tablespoons
    water
Chopped fresh parsley

□ In large nonstick skillet over medium-high heat, heat oil. Add onion, red pepper and garlic and cook, stirring frequently, 4 minutes or until soft. Add water, vinegar, sugar, sherry, soy sauce and pepper; bring to a boil. Add fillets, cover and simmer 10 minutes or until fish flakes easily. With slotted spatula, transfer fillets to serving platter; keep warm.

Add cornstarch mixture to skillet. Cook, stirring constantly, 1 minute or until thickened. Pour over fillets. Sprinkle with parsley. **MAKES 4 SERVINGS**, about 3 ounces fish each.

APPROXIMATE NUTRIENT ANALYSIS PER SERVING:

Calories □ 225
Protein □ 17 grams
Fat □ 4 grams
Carbohydrate □ 12 grams
Cholesterol □ 68 milligrams
Sodium □ 95 milligrams
Potassium □ 25 milligrams

% Calories from Fat □ 22
% Calories from Saturated Fat
    □ 4.5
% Calories from
    Monounsaturated Fat □ 6.5
% Calories from Polyunsaturated
    Fat □ 11
P/S □ 2.6

*Thin chicken cutlets may be substituted for fish fillets. Increase cooking time by about 10 minutes.

FOOD GROUP UNITS:

Grains □ ⅓   Fat:
Meat and Alternatives: Polyunsaturated □ ½
   Very Low-Fat □ 2

SALMON LOAF

1 can (15½ ounces) low-   ¼ cup skim milk
   sodium salmon in water,   2 tablespoons minced onion
   drained and flaked (2 cups)   1 tablespoon fresh lemon
1 cup fresh whole-wheat   juice
   bread crumbs (2 slices)   ½ teaspoon dried dill weed
1 cup cooked rice   ⅛ teaspoon ground black
1 egg, slightly beaten   pepper
1 egg white, slightly beaten

□ Preheat oven to 375°F. In large bowl, combine all ingredients; mix well. Spray 9- × 5-inch loaf pan with nonstick cooking spray. Spoon mixture into pan, pressing down lightly. Bake 45 minutes or until knife inserted in center comes out clean. Invert onto serving platter. MAKES 8 SERVINGS.

APPROXIMATE NUTRIENT ANALYSIS PER SERVING:

Calories □ 135   % Calories from Fat □ 32
Protein □ 14 grams   % Calories from Saturated Fat
Fat □ 5 grams   □ 8
Carbohydrate □ 10 grams   % Calories from
Cholesterol □ 76 milligrams   Monounsaturated Fat □ 16
Sodium □ 100 milligrams   % Calories from Polyunsaturated
Potassium □ 250 milligrams   Fat □ 8
                                 P/S □ 1.1

FOOD GROUP UNITS:

Grains □ ½
Meat and Alternatives:
   Very Low-Fat □ 2

LEMON-BREAD STUFFED FISH

1 tablespoon unsalted margarine
¼ cup chopped onion
¼ cup chopped celery
1 garlic clove, minced
1½ cups fresh whole-wheat bread crumbs (3 slices)
2 tablespoons chopped fresh parsley

2 tablespoons fresh lemon juice, divided
1 tablespoon dry white wine
½ teaspoon grated lemon peel
¼ teaspoon dried thyme
⅛ teaspoon ground black pepper
1½ pounds pan-dressed fish (trout or striped bass), head and tail removed

□ Preheat oven to 350°F. Spray baking dish with nonstick cooking spray or line with foil. In medium-size saucepan over medium-high heat, melt margarine. Add onion, celery and garlic and cook 4 minutes or until soft. Remove from heat. Stir in bread crumbs, parsley, 1 tablespoon lemon juice, wine, lemon peel, thyme and pepper. Fill cavity of fish with stuffing, securing with toothpicks or skewers; place in baking dish. Sprinkle with remaining lemon juice; cover. Bake 40 minutes or until fish flakes. MAKES 4 SERVINGS.

APPROXIMATE NUTRIENT ANALYSIS PER SERVING:

Calories □ 370
Protein □ 28 grams
Fat □ 7 grams
Carbohydrate □ 21 grams
Cholesterol □ 102 milligrams
Sodium □ 215 milligrams
Potassium □ 95 milligrams

% Calories from Fat □ 24
% Calories from Saturated Fat □ 6
% Calories from Monounsaturated Fat □ 9
% Calories from Polyunsaturated Fat □ 9
P/S □ 1.6

FOOD GROUP UNITS:

Grains □ 1
Meat and Alternatives:
Very Low-Fat □ 3½

Fat:
Polyunsaturated □ ½

Mexican Baked Fish

1 tablespoon vegetable oil
¼ cup chopped onion
2 garlic cloves, minced
1 can (16 ounces) tomatoes, canned without salt, drained and chopped
1 tablespoon chopped green chilies
1 teaspoon chili powder

⅛ teaspoon ground black pepper
1 egg white
1 tablespoon skim milk
½ cup cornmeal
4 flounder fillets (1 pound)
2 ounces shredded part-skim mozzarella cheese (½ cup)

□ Preheat oven to 350°F. In small saucepan over medium-high heat, heat oil. Add onion and garlic and cook, stirring frequently, 3 minutes or until soft. Add tomatoes, chilies, chili powder and pepper; bring to a boil. Reduce heat, cover and simmer, stirring occasionally, about 15 minutes.

In shallow dish, beat egg white and skim milk slightly. Place cornmeal on waxed paper. Dip fillets in egg mixture; coat in cornmeal. Spray baking dish with nonstick cooking spray. Place fillets in dish in single layer. Pour sauce over fish; sprinkle with cheese. Bake 20 minutes or until fish flakes. MAKES 4 SERVINGS, about 3 ounces fish each.

APPROXIMATE NUTRIENT ANALYSIS PER SERVING:

Calories □ 335
Protein □ 33 grams
Fat □ 7 grams
Carbohydrate □ 21 grams
Cholesterol □ 51 milligrams
Sodium □ 305 milligrams
Potassium □ 840 milligrams

% Calories from Fat □ 18
% Calories from Saturated Fat
□ 6
% Calories from
Monounsaturated Fat □ 5
% Calories from Polyunsaturated
Fat □ 7
P/S □ 1.2

Food Group Units:

Vegetables □ 1
Grains □ 1
Meat and Alternatives:
Very Low-Fat □ 3½

Fat:
Polyunsaturated □ ½

CHICKEN ENCHILADAS

3 teaspoons vegetable oil,
divided
2 garlic cloves, minced
1 can (16 ounces) tomatoes,
canned without salt,
chopped
3 teaspoons chili powder,
divided
⅛ teaspoon ground black
pepper
1½ cups chopped cooked
chicken (about 8 ounces
cooked)

¼ cup plain low-fat yogurt
3 tablespoons chopped green
chilies
2 tablespoons finely chopped
green onion
4 corn tortillas
2 ounces shredded part-skim
mozzarella cheese

□ In medium-size saucepan over medium heat, heat 2 teaspoons oil. Add garlic and cook about 1 minute. Add tomatoes, 2 teaspoons chili powder and pepper; simmer uncovered, stirring occasionally, about 30 minutes.

Meanwhile, in small bowl, combine chicken, yogurt, green chilies, green onion and remaining chili powder; mix well.

In large nonstick skillet, heat remaining oil. Add tortillas, one at a time. Cook 1 minute on each side or until soft.

Meanwhile, preheat oven to 350°F. Spoon ¼ cup sauce into 8-inch square baking dish. Spread an equal amount of chicken mixture in center of each tortilla. Fold sides over filling. Place tortilla seam-side down in baking dish. Pour sauce over tortillas. Sprinkle with cheese. Bake 30 minutes or until heated through. MAKES 4 SERVINGS.

APPROXIMATE NUTRIENT ANALYSIS PER SERVING:

Calories □ 270
Protein □ 26 grams
Fat □ 10 grams

% Calories from Fat □ 32
% Calories from Saturated Fat
□ 11

Carbohydrate ◻ 21 grams
Cholesterol ◻ 57 milligrams
Sodium ◻ 205 milligrams
Potassium ◻ 560 milligrams

% Calories from
  Monounsaturated Fat ◻ 10
% Calories from Polyunsaturated
  Fat ◻ 11
P/S ◻ 1.0

FOOD GROUP UNITS:

Vegetables ◻ 1
Grains ◻ 1
Meat and Alternatives:
  Very Low-Fat ◻ 2½
  Moderately Low-Fat ◻ ½

Fat:
  Polyunsaturated ◻ 1

CHICKEN BUNDLES

2 whole chicken breasts, split,
  skinned and boned (1
  pound boneless)
3 teaspoons unsalted
  margarine, divided
2 tablespoons finely chopped
  onion
1 cup mashed sweet potatoes
  (about 2)
2 tablespoons dry white wine
2 teaspoons honey

½ teaspoon grated orange
  peel
⅛ teaspoon ground cinnamon
Dash ground nutmeg
Dash ground black pepper
2 tablespoons wheat bran

◻ Preheat oven to 400°F. On cutting board with meat
mallet, pound chicken to ¼-inch thickness; set aside.

In small skillet over medium heat, melt 1 teaspoon
margarine. Add onion and cook 3 minutes or until soft. Stir
in sweet potato, wine, honey, orange peel, cinnamon,
nutmeg and pepper; cook about 1 minute.

Spoon mixture by tablespoonsful onto each chicken
breast; roll up and secure with toothpicks. Place roll-ups
seam-side down in 8-inch square baking dish. Cover and
bake 20 minutes or until chicken is tender.

Meanwhile, in small saucepan over medium heat, melt remaining margarine. Sprinkle bundles with wheat bran; drizzle melted margarine over top. Increase oven heat to broil. Broil chicken 3 to 4 inches from heat 1 minute, until browned.

APPROXIMATE NUTRIENT ANALYSIS PER SERVING:

Calories □ 280
Protein □ 29 grams
Fat □ 6 grams
Carbohydrate □ 26 grams
Cholesterol □ 73 milligrams
Sodium □ 75 milligrams
Potassium □ 380 milligrams

% Calories from Fat □ 21
% Calories from Saturated Fat □ 5.5
% Calories from Monounsaturated Fat □ 9
% Calories from Polyunsaturated Fat □ 6.5
P/S □ 1.1

FOOD GROUP UNITS:

Vegetables □ 1
Grains □ 1
Meat and Alternatives:
    Very Low-Fat □ 3

Fat:
    Polyunsaturated □ ½

CHICKEN AND VEGETABLES IN CREAM SAUCE

2 whole chicken breasts, split, skinned and boned (1 pound boneless)
1 tablespoon canola oil
½ cup chopped onion
1 large garlic clove, minced
1 cup julienne carrots (3 medium)
1 cup julienne zucchini (1 medium)
½ teaspoon dried basil
½ teaspoon dried thyme

1 cup low-sodium chicken broth
¼ teaspoon ground black pepper
⅛ teaspoon salt
1 large tomato, peeled, seeded, cut into thin strips
¼ cup low-fat milk
2 teaspoons Dijon-style mustard
2 cups cooked brown rice (keep warm)

□ Spray a large nonstick skillet with nonstick cooking spray and heat over medium-high heat. Add chicken cutlets and brown 2 to 3 minutes on each side; remove to a platter. Add oil to skillet and sauté onion and garlic, stirring frequently, 2 to 3 minutes. Add carrots, zucchini, basil and thyme. Sauté, stirring frequently, 2 minutes. Return chicken to skillet with chicken broth, pepper and salt. Reduce heat to medium, cover and simmer 10 minutes, turning chicken once. With slotted spoon, remove chicken and vegetables to serving platter and keep warm. Add tomato, milk and mustard to skillet. Increase heat to high and cook, stirring, until sauce is slightly thickened. Spoon over chicken. Serve with brown rice. MAKES 4 SERVINGS.

APPROXIMATE NUTRIENT ANALYSIS PER SERVING:

Calories □ 355
Protein □ 35 grams
Fat □ 9 grams
Carbohydrate □ 36 grams
Cholesterol □ 74 milligrams
Sodium □ 270 milligrams
Potassium □ 680 milligrams

% Calories from Fat □ 29
% Calories from Saturated Fat
□ 7
% Calories from
Monounsaturated Fat □ 13
% Calories from Polyunsaturated
Fat □ 9
P/S □ 1.3

FOOD GROUP UNITS:

Grains □ 1
Vegetables □ 2
Meat and Alternatives:
Very Low-Fat □ 4

Fat:
Monounsaturated □ 1

CHICKEN AND VEGETABLE STIR FRY

⅓ cup low-sodium chicken broth
2 tablespoons sherry
1 tablespoon low-sodium soy sauce
1 tablespoon cornstarch
⅛ teaspoon ground black pepper
2 whole chicken breasts, split, skinned and boned (1 pound boneless), cut into ½-inch pieces

1 tablespoon peanut oil
1 package (6 ounces) frozen snow peas, thawed and well drained
¼ pound mushrooms, sliced (1½ cups)
2 tablespoons chopped green onion
2 garlic cloves, minced
¼ teaspoon finely chopped fresh ginger

□ In shallow dish, combine chicken broth, sherry, soy sauce, cornstarch and pepper. Add chicken; toss well. Cover and refrigerate, stirring occasionally, about 1 hour.

In large nonstick skillet over high heat, heat oil. Add snow peas, mushrooms, green onion, garlic and ginger and cook 3 to 5 minutes or until tender-crisp. Remove from skillet; set aside.

Add chicken with marinade to skillet; cook, stirring occasionally, 10 minutes or until chicken is tender and sauce is thickened. If necessary, add about ¼ cup water to skillet.

Return vegetables to skillet; cook, stirring frequently, about 1 minute. MAKES 4 SERVINGS, about ¾ cup each.

APPROXIMATE NUTRIENT ANALYSIS PER SERVING:

Calories □ 215
Protein □ 30 grams
Fat □ 7 grams

% Calories from Fat □ 21
% Calories from Saturated Fat □ 5

Carbohydrate □ 8 grams
Cholesterol □ 73 milligrams
Sodium □ 225 milligrams
Potassium □ 440 milligrams

% Calories from
Monounsaturated Fat □ 10
% Calories from Polyunsaturated
Fat □ 6
P/S □ 1.2

FOOD GROUP UNITS:

Vegetables □ 2
Meat and Alternatives:
Very Low-Fat □ 3

Fat:
Monounsaturated □ 1

ORANGE CHICKEN

1 tablespoon vegetable oil
2 whole chicken breasts, split, skinned and boned (1 pound boneless)
1 cup red pepper, cut into chunks (1 medium)
2 tablespoons chopped green onion
1 garlic clove, minced
¾ cup orange juice

1 teaspoon prepared mustard
¼ teaspoon salt
⅛ teaspoon ground black pepper
2 teaspoons cornstarch dissolved in 2 tablespoons water
½ cup fresh orange sections, cut into bite-size pieces (½ medium)
Fresh parsley for garnish

□ In large nonstick skillet over medium-high heat, heat oil. Add chicken and brown. Remove from skillet. Add red pepper, green onion and garlic and cook, stirring occasionally, 5 minutes or until tender.

Return chicken to skillet. Add orange juice, mustard, salt and pepper; bring to a boil. Reduce heat, cover and simmer about 20 minutes. Transfer chicken to serving platter; keep warm.

Add cornstarch mixture to skillet. Increase heat to high; add orange sections. Cook, stirring frequently, 1 to 2 minutes or until thickened. Pour over chicken. Garnish with parsley. **MAKES 4 SERVINGS**, about 3 ounces chicken each.

APPROXIMATE NUTRIENT ANALYSIS PER SERVING:

Calories □ 220
Protein □ 28 grams
Fat □ 7 grams
Carbohydrate □ 11 grams
Cholesterol □ 73 milligrams
Sodium □ 205 milligrams
Potassium □ 445 milligrams

% Calories from Fat □ 28
% Calories from Saturated Fat
 □ 7
% Calories from
 Monounsaturated Fat □ 9
% Calories from Polyunsaturated
 Fat □ 12
P/S □ 2.1

FOOD GROUP UNITS:

Vegetables □ 2
Fruits □ 1
Meat and Alternatives:
 Very Low-Fat □ 3

Fat:
 Polyunsaturated □ ½

CHICKEN DIVAN

4 whole chicken breasts, split, skinned and boned (1 pound boneless, raw)
1 package (10 ounces) frozen broccoli spears, cooked and drained (or 2 cups fresh, steamed)
2 tablespoons unsalted margarine
¼ cup chopped onion
¼ cup all-purpose flour

1½ cups skim milk
2 tablespoons dry sherry
⅛ teaspoon ground black pepper
Dash ground nutmeg
1½ tablespoons freshly grated Parmesan cheese

□ Preheat oven to 400°F. Spray nonstick skillet with nonstick cooking spray. Over medium-high heat, brown chicken breasts. Arrange broccoli in 8-inch square baking pan. Place chicken in single layer over broccoli.

In medium-size saucepan over low heat, or in double boiler, melt margarine. Add onion and cook, stirring frequently, about 3 minutes. Stir in flour; cook, stirring constantly, about 1 minute. Gradually add milk, sherry, pepper and nutmeg. Cook, stirring constantly, until thickened and smooth. Pour over chicken and broccoli. Sprinkle with cheese. Bake 20 minutes or until bubbly. MAKES 4 SERVINGS, about 3 ounces chicken each.

APPROXIMATE NUTRIENT ANALYSIS PER SERVING:

Calories □ 430
Protein □ 61 grams
Fat □ 13 grams
Carbohydrate □ 15 grams
Cholesterol □ 149 milligrams
Sodium □ 235 milligrams
Potassium □ 750 milligrams

% Calories from Fat □ 28
% Calories from Saturated Fat
   □ 8.5
% Calories from
   Monounsaturated Fat □ 12
% Calories from Polyunsaturated
   Fat □ 7.5
P/S □ 0.1

FOOD GROUP UNITS:

Vegetables □ 1
Grains □ ½
Meat and Alternatives:
   Very Low-Fat □ 3
Milk Products:
   Very Low-Fat □ ½

Fat:
   Polyunsaturated □ 1

CHICKEN WITH CURRANT SAUCE

2 whole chicken breasts, split,
   skinned and boned (1
   pound boneless)
1 tablespoon margarine
2 tablespoons finely chopped
   onion
1 garlic clove, minced
½ cup currant jelly

¼ cup raisins
⅛ teaspoon dry mustard
   powder
⅛ teaspoon salt
⅛ teaspoon ground black
   pepper
2 teaspoons cornstarch
   dissolved in 2 tablespoons
   water

□ Preheat oven to 400°F. Spray 8-inch square baking dish with nonstick cooking spray. Place chicken in dish. Cover; bake 20 to 30 minutes or until tender.

Meanwhile, in small saucepan over medium heat, melt margarine. Add onion and garlic and cook 3 minutes or until soft. Add jelly, raisins, mustard, salt and pepper. Cook, stirring constantly, until jelly is melted.

Add cornstarch mixture to saucepan; cook, stirring constantly, until thickened. Serve sauce with chicken. MAKES 4 SERVINGS, about 3 ounces chicken each.

APPROXIMATE NUTRIENT ANALYSIS PER SERVING:

Calories □ 305
Protein □ 30 grams
Fat □ 6 grams
Carbohydrate □ 36 grams
Cholesterol □ 73 milligrams
Sodium □ 180 milligrams
Potassium □ 340 milligrams

% Calories from Fat □ 18
% Calories from Saturated Fat
  □ 5
% Calories from
  Monounsaturated Fat □ 7
% Calories from Polyunsaturated
  Fat □ 6
P/S □ 1.3

FOOD GROUP UNITS:

Fruits □ 1
Grains □ 1½
Meat and Alternatives:
  Very Low-Fat □ 3

Fat:
  Polyunsaturated □ 1

CHICKEN WITH WINE SAUCE

1 tablespoon vegetable oil
2 whole chicken breasts, split, skinned and boned (1 pound boneless)
½ pound mushrooms, sliced (3½ cups)
¼ cup chopped onion
2 garlic cloves, minced
½ cup dry red wine

⅓ cup + 1½ tablespoons water, divided
¼ teaspoon dried thyme
¼ teaspoon salt
⅛ teaspoon ground black pepper
2 teaspoons all-purpose flour
2 tablespoons chopped fresh parsley

□ In large nonstick skillet over medium heat, heat oil. Add chicken and brown. Remove from skillet. Add mushrooms, onion and garlic to drippings in skillet. Cook, stirring occasionally, 5 minutes or until tender. Return chicken to skillet. Add red wine, ⅓ cup water, thyme, salt and pepper; bring to a boil. Reduce heat, cover and simmer, turning once, about 20 minutes or until chicken is tender. Transfer chicken to serving platter; keep warm.

In small bowl, combine flour and remaining 1½ tablespoons water; add to skillet. Cook, stirring constantly, about 1 minute. Stir in parsley. Spoon sauce over chicken. MAKES 4 SERVINGS.

APPROXIMATE NUTRIENT ANALYSIS PER SERVING:

Calories □ 200
Protein □ 20 grams
Fat □ 7 grams
Carbohydrate □ 5 grams
Cholesterol □ 73 milligrams
Sodium □ 190 milligrams
Potassium □ 470 milligrams

% Calories from Fat □ 31
% Calories from Saturated Fat
 □ 8.5
% Calories from
 Monounsaturated Fat □ 10
% Calories from Polyunsaturated
 Fat □ 12.5
P/S □ 1.6

FOOD GROUP UNITS:

Vegetables □ 1
Meat and Alternatives:
 Very Low-Fat □ 3

Fat:
 Polyunsaturated □ 1

SPICY CHICKEN WINGS

2 pounds chicken wings,
halved and skinned (about
12-16)
¾ cup plain low-fat yogurt
1 tablespoon vegetable oil
1 tablespoon dry sherry
1 garlic clove, minced
½ teaspoon finely chopped
fresh ginger

½ teaspoon grated orange
peel
⅛ teaspoon ground red
pepper
1½ cups crushed unsalted,
whole-grain crackers (about
36)
¼ cup toasted sesame seeds

□ Place chicken wings in shallow dish. In small bowl,
combine yogurt, oil, sherry, garlic, ginger, orange peel
and red pepper. Pour over wings; toss well. Cover and
refrigerate, stirring occasionally, about 2 hours.

Preheat oven to 375°F. Spray baking pan with nonstick
cooking spray. In shallow dish, combine cracker crumbs
and sesame seeds. Coat chicken wings evenly with crumb
mixture; place on baking pan. Bake about 30 minutes.
MAKES 4 SERVINGS.

APPROXIMATE NUTRIENT ANALYSIS PER SERVING:

Calories □ 340
Protein □ 26 grams
Fat □ 18 grams
Carbohydrate □ 16 grams
Cholesterol □ 65 milligrams
Sodium □ 138 milligrams
Potassium □ 331 milligrams

% Calories from Fat □ 49
% Calories from Saturated Fat
□ 19
% Calories from
Monounsaturated Fat □ 14
% Calories from Polyunsaturated
Fat □ 16
P/S □ 0.8

FOOD GROUP UNITS:

Grains □ 1
Meat and Alternatives:
Very Low-Fat □ 3
Milk Products:
Moderately Low-Fat □ ¼

Fat:
Polyunsaturated □ 1½

Chicken and Lima Bean Casserole

2 packages (10 ounces each)
frozen lima beans
1½ cups cooked, cubed
chicken (9 ounces cooked)
1 can (16 ounces) tomatoes,
canned without salt,
drained and chopped
¼ cup finely chopped onion
1 garlic clove, minced

1½ teaspoons dry mustard
powder
1 teaspoon Worcestershire
sauce
⅛ teaspoon ground black
pepper
4 ounces shredded part-skim
mozzarella cheese (1 cup)
¼ cup fresh whole-wheat
bread crumbs

□ Preheat oven to 375°F. Prepare beans according to package directions but without salt. Spray 1½-quart baking dish with nonstick cooking spray. Place beans in dish.

In large bowl, combine chicken, tomatoes, onion, garlic, mustard, Worcestershire sauce and pepper; mix well. Pour mixture over beans. Sprinkle cheese and bread crumbs over bean mixture. Bake 30 minutes or until hot and bubbly. MAKES 6 SERVINGS.

APPROXIMATE NUTRIENT ANALYSIS PER SERVING:

Calories □ 240
Protein □ 25 grams
Fat □ 5 grams
Carbohydrate □ 24 grams
Cholesterol □ 47 milligrams
Sodium □ 200 milligrams
Potassium □ 700 milligrams

% Calories from Fat □ 20
% Calories from Saturated Fat
□ 10
% Calories from
Monounsaturated Fat □ 6.5
% Calories from Polyunsaturated
Fat □ 3.5
P/S □ 0.3

Food Group Units:

Vegetables □ 1
Legumes □ 1
Meat and Alternatives:
    Very Low-Fat □ 1½
    Moderate Fat □ ½

TURKEY TETRAZZINI

4 ounces spaghetti (2 cups cooked)
1 tablespoon unsalted margarine
¼ pound mushrooms, sliced (1½ cups)
2 tablespoons chopped onion
2 tablespoons all-purpose flour
1½ cups skim milk

1 tablespoon sherry
⅛ teaspoon ground black pepper
⅛ teaspoon ground nutmeg
1½ cups cooked, cubed turkey or chicken (9 ounces cooked)
2 tablespoons chopped pimento
2 tablespoons freshly grated Parmesan cheese

□ Preheat oven to 350°F. Cook spaghetti according to package directions but without salt.

Meanwhile, in small saucepan over medium-high heat, melt margarine. Add mushrooms and onion and cook, stirring occasionally, about 4 minutes. Add flour and cook, stirring constantly, about 1 minute. Gradually add milk, sherry, pepper and nutmeg and cook, stirring constantly, 5 minutes or until thickened.

Spray 1-quart casserole dish with nonstick cooking spray. Place spaghetti, turkey, pimento and sauce in dish; toss well. Sprinkle with cheese, cover. Bake 20 to 25 minutes or until hot and bubbly. **MAKES 4 SERVINGS.**

APPROXIMATE NUTRIENT ANALYSIS PER SERVING:

Calories □ 275
Protein □ 25 grams
Fat □ 6 grams
Carbohydrate □ 29 grams
Cholesterol □ 40 milligrams
Sodium □ 140 milligrams
Potassium □ 495 milligrams

% Calories from Fat □ 21
% Calories from Saturated Fat □ 7.5
% Calories from Monounsaturated Fat □ 7.5
% Calories from Polyunsaturated Fat □ 6
P/S □ 0.8

FOOD GROUP UNITS:

Vegetables □ 1
Grains □ 1½
Meat and Alternatives:
    Very Low-Fat □ 2½
Milk Products:
    Very Low-Fat □ ½

Fat:
    Polyunsaturated □ 1

TURKEY LOAF

1½ pounds ground turkey
1 cup fresh whole wheat
    bread crumbs (2 slices)
½ cup chopped onion
¼ cup chopped celery
¼ cup chopped green pepper
¼ cup chopped fresh parsley
¼ cup skim milk

2 garlic cloves, minced
1 large egg, slightly beaten
¾ teaspoon dried dill weed
½ teaspoon grated lemon peel
½ teaspoon ground sage
⅛ teaspoon ground black
    pepper

□ Preheat oven to 350°F. Spray 9- × 5-inch loaf pan with nonstick cooking spray. In large bowl, mix all ingredients; blend well. Spoon into pan and shape into a loaf. Bake 50 to 60 minutes or until loaf pulls away from sides of pan. Remove to serving platter. Cool 10 minutes before slicing. **MAKES 6 SERVINGS.**

APPROXIMATE NUTRIENT ANALYSIS PER SERVING:

Calories □ 210
Protein □ 23 grams
Fat □ 10 grams
Carbohydrate □ 7 grams
Cholesterol □ 128 milligrams
Sodium □ 185 milligrams
Potassium □ 115 milligrams

% Calories from Fat □ 43
% Calories from Saturated Fat
    □ 14
% Calories from
    Monounsaturated Fat □ 17
% Calories from Polyunsaturated
    Fat □ 12
P/S □ 0.8

FOOD GROUP UNITS:

Grains □ ½
Meat and Alternatives:
    Very Low-Fat □ 3

VEAL STEW

1½ pounds veal stew meat,
cut into 1-inch pieces
2 tablespoons all-purpose
flour
2 tablespoons margarine
2 small onions, peeled and
cut into quarters
1 garlic clove, minced
1½ cups low-sodium beef
broth
½ cup dry white wine

1 bay leaf
½ teaspoon dried thyme
⅛ teaspoon salt
⅛ teaspoon ground black
pepper
4 carrots, peeled and cut in
chunks
2 small potatoes, peeled and
cut in chunks
½ cup water

□ In plastic bag, combine meat and flour; toss to coat. In large saucepan over medium-high heat, melt margarine. Add veal and brown. Reduce heat to medium; add onions and garlic to drippings in saucepan. Cook, stirring occasionally, 5 minutes or until soft.

Add beef broth, wine, bay leaf, thyme, salt and pepper; bring to a boil. Reduce heat, cover and simmer about 1¼ hours. Add carrots, potatoes and water; continue to simmer 45 minutes or until meat and vegetables are tender.

Increase heat to medium-high, remove cover and cook 10 minutes. Remove and discard bay leaf. MAKES 6 SERVINGS, about 1 cup each.

APPROXIMATE NUTRIENT ANALYSIS PER SERVING:

Calories □ 155
Protein □ 8 grams
Fat □ 7 grams
Carbohydrate □ 17 grams
Cholesterol □ 22 milligrams
Sodium □ 125 milligrams
Potassium □ 815 milligrams

% Calories from Fat □ 38
% Calories from Saturated Fat
□ 12
% Calories from
Monounsaturated Fat □ 15
% Calories from Polyunsaturated
Fat □ 11
P/S □ 1.0

FOOD GROUP UNITS:

Vegetables □ ½   Fat:
Grains □ ½   Polyunsaturated □ 1
Meat and Alternatives:
  Very Low-Fat □ 1

VEAL CHOPS WITH MUSHROOMS

4 veal rib chops, about ¾-inch thick (2 pounds)
1 tablespoon unsalted margarine
¼ cup chopped onion
1 garlic clove, minced
½ pound mushrooms, sliced (3 cups)

1 can (16 ounces) tomatoes, canned without salt, chopped
2 tablespoons dry red wine
¼ teaspoon dried rosemary
⅛ teaspoon ground black pepper

□ Trim fat from chops. Spray large nonstick skillet with nonstick cooking spray. In skillet over medium-high heat, brown chops. Remove from skillet.

Add margarine, onion and garlic to skillet. Cook, stirring occasionally, 3 minutes or until soft. Add mushrooms and cook, stirring occasionally, about 5 minutes. Add tomatoes and their juice, wine, rosemary and pepper; bring to a boil. Reduce heat; return chops to skillet. Cover and simmer, turning occasionally, 45 minutes or until veal is tender. Transfer chops to serving platter; keep warm.

Increase heat to high. Cook, stirring frequently, 5 to 7 minutes or until reduced and slightly thickened. Spoon sauce over chops. MAKES 4 SERVINGS, about 4 ounces of veal each.

APPROXIMATE NUTRIENT ANALYSIS PER SERVING:

Calories □ 300
Protein □ 26 grams
Fat □ 17 grams

% Calories from Fat □ 53
% Calories from Saturated Fat
  □ 21

Carbohydrate □ 9 grams
Cholesterol □ 87 milligrams
Sodium □ 85 milligrams
Potassium □ 740 milligrams

% Calories from
  Monounsaturated Fat □ 23
% Calories from Polyunsaturated
  Fat □ 9
P/S □ 0.4

FOOD GROUP UNITS:

Vegetables □ 2
Meat and Alternatives:
  Very Low-Fat □ 4

Fat:
  Polyunsaturated □ 1

VEAL PICCATA

4 veal cutlets, about ¼-inch
  thick (1 pound)
2 tablespoons all-purpose
  flour
2 teaspoons margarine
1 teaspoon olive oil
1 garlic clove, minced
¼ cup chopped fresh parsley

1 tablespoon fresh lemon
  juice
⅛ teaspoon grated lemon peel
¼ teaspoon salt
⅛ teaspoon ground black
  pepper
2 tablespoons water

□ On cutting board with meat mallet, pound veal cutlets to ⅛-inch thickness. Coat with flour, shaking off excess. In large nonstick skillet over medium-high heat, heat margarine and oil. Add cutlets and brown. Remove from skillet.

Add remaining ingredients, except water, to skillet. Cook, stirring frequently, about 2 minutes. Return veal to skillet; add water. Reduce heat, cover and simmer 10 to 15 minutes or until veal is tender. **MAKES 4 SERVINGS.**

APPROXIMATE NUTRIENT ANALYSIS PER SERVING:

Calories □ 230
Protein □ 24 grams
Fat □ 12 grams

% Calories from Fat □ 50
% Calories from Saturated Fat
  □ 20

Carbohydrate □ 4 grams
Cholesterol □ 87 milligrams
Sodium □ 220 milligrams
Potassium □ 295 milligrams

% Calories from
  Monounsaturated Fat □ 24
% Calories from Polyunsaturated
  Fat □ 6
P/S □ 0.3

FOOD GROUP UNITS:

Vegetables □ 1
Meat and Alternatives:
  Very Low-Fat □ 3

Fat:
  Polyunsaturated □ 1

STUFFED VEAL ROLLS

4 veal cutlets, about ¼-inch
  thick (1 pound)
1 tablespoon unsalted
  margarine
¼ cup finely chopped carrots
¼ cup finely chopped celery
2 tablespoons finely chopped
  onion
1 garlic clove, minced
1 cup cooked brown rice

1 tablespoon chopped fresh
  parsley
¼ teaspoon dried sage
¼ teaspoon ground black
  pepper
1 cup low-sodium beef broth
¼ pound mushrooms, sliced
  (about ½ cup)
2 teaspoons flour
2 tablespoons water

□ On cutting board with meat mallet, pound veal cutlets
to ⅛-inch thickness; set aside.

In small saucepan over medium-high heat, melt margarine. Add carrots, celery, onion and garlic and cook, stirring occasionally, 5 minutes or until tender. Remove from
heat; stir in rice, parsley and seasonings.

With tablespoon, spoon an equal amount of stuffing onto
each veal cutlet; roll up and secure with toothpicks.

Spray large nonstick skillet with nonstick cooking spray.
Over medium heat, brown veal rolls on all sides. Add beef
broth and mushrooms; bring to a boil. Reduce heat; cover.
Add any leftover stuffing to skillet. Simmer 20 to 30

minutes or until veal is fork tender. Transfer veal to serving platter; keep warm.

In small bowl, combine flour and water; mix well. Add to liquid in skillet; cook, stirring constantly, until thickened. Pour over veal. MAKES 4 SERVINGS, about 3 ounces veal each.

APPROXIMATE NUTRIENT ANALYSIS PER SERVING:

Calories □ 290
Protein □ 26 grams
Fat □ 12 grams
Carbohydrate □ 17 grams
Cholesterol □ 90 milligrams
Sodium □ 80 milligrams
Potassium □ 620 milligrams

% Calories from Fat □ 39
% Calories from Saturated Fat
□ 15
% Calories from
Monounsaturated Fat □ 17
% Calories from Polyunsaturated
Fat □ 7
P/S □ 0.3

FOOD GROUP UNITS:

Vegetables □ ½
Grains □ ½
Meat and Alternatives:
Very Low-Fat □ 3

Fat:
Polyunsaturated □ ½

VEAL PARMIGIANA

4 veal cutlets, about ¼-inch thick (1 pound)
½ cup plain dry bread crumbs
2¼ teaspoons freshly grated Parmesan cheese
1 egg
1 tablespoon water

1 tablespoon olive oil
1½ cups no-salt-added spaghetti sauce
½ cup shredded part-skim mozzarella cheese (2 ounces)
¼ teaspoon dried oregano

□ Preheat oven to 375°F. On cutting board with meat mallet, pound veal cutlets to ⅛-inch thickness. In shallow dish, combine bread crumbs and Parmesan cheese; mix well. In another shallow dish, beat egg and water slightly. Dip veal into egg mixture, then coat with bread-crumb mixture.

In large nonstick skillet over medium-high heat, heat oil. Add veal and brown. Arrange cutlets in single layer in shallow 2-quart baking dish. Pour sauce over veal. Sprinkle with mozzarella cheese and oregano.

Bake 20 to 30 minutes or until bubbly. MAKES 4 SERVINGS, about 4 ounces veal each.

APPROXIMATE NUTRIENT ANALYSIS PER SERVING:

Calories □ 380
Protein □ 32 grams
Fat □ 19 grams
Carbohydrate □ 17 grams
Cholesterol □ 165 milligrams
Sodium □ 300 milligrams
Potassium □ 310 milligrams

% Calories from Fat □ 46
% Calories from Saturated Fat
□ 18
% Calories from
Monounsaturated Fat □ 22
% Calories from Polyunsaturated
Fat □ 6
P/S □ 0.1

FOOD GROUP UNITS:

Vegetables □ 1
Meat and Alternatives:
    Very Low-Fat □ 3
    Moderately Low-Fat □ 1

Fat:
    Monounsaturated □ 1

VEAL AND PEPPERS

4 veal cutlets, about ¼-inch
    thick (1 pound)
1½ tablespoons olive oil
1½ cups green pepper strips
    (1 large)
1½ cups red pepper strips (1
    large)
½ cup sliced onion

2 garlic cloves, minced
¼ cup dry white wine
¼ teaspoon salt
¼ teaspoon dried sage
⅛ teaspoon ground black
    pepper

□ On cutting board with meat mallet, pound veal cutlets
to ⅛-inch thickness. Cut into ½-inch strips. In large nonstick skillet over medium-high heat, heat oil. Add veal and
brown. Remove from skillet. Reduce heat to medium; add
red and green peppers, onion and garlic. Cook, stirring
occasionally, 7 minutes or until soft.

Return veal to skillet; add remaining ingredients. Cook,
stirring occasionally, 15 to 20 minutes or until tender. If
necessary, add 1 to 2 tablespoons water. MAKES 4 SERV-
INGS, about 3 ounces veal each.

APPROXIMATE NUTRIENT ANALYSIS PER SERVING:

Calories □ 255
Protein □ 24 grams
Fat □ 14 grams
Carbohydrate □ 6 grams
Cholesterol □ 87 milligrams
Sodium □ 200 milligrams
Potassium □ 455 milligrams

% Calories from Fat □ 52
% Calories from Saturated Fat
    □ 18
% Calories from
    Monounsaturated Fat □ 28
% Calories from Polyunsaturated
    Fat □ 6
P/S □ 0.2

FOOD GROUP UNITS:

Vegetables □ 2
Meat and Alternatives:
    Very Low-Fat □ 3

Fat:
    Monounsaturated □ 1

MOUSSAKA

1½-1¾ pounds eggplant, peeled and sliced ¼ inch thick (1½ medium)
1 pound ground lamb, trimmed of visible fat before grinding
½ cup chopped onion
2 garlic cloves, minced
½ cup low-sodium tomato sauce
¼ cup dry red wine
½ teaspoon dried oregano
¼ teaspoon ground black pepper, divided
¼ teaspoon ground cinnamon
3 tablespoons all-purpose flour, divided
2 tablespoons water
1 tablespoon unsalted margarine
1½ cups skim milk
1 tablespoon freshly grated Parmesan cheese

□ Spray large nonstick skillet with nonstick cooking spray. In skillet, brown eggplant slices; set aside. In same skillet, brown lamb. Drain and discard excess fat. Add onion and garlic to skillet. Cook, stirring frequently, about 3 minutes. Add tomato sauce, wine, oregano, ⅛ teaspoon pepper and cinnamon; cook, stirring occasionally, about 20 minutes.

In small bowl, combine 1 tablespoon flour and water. Add to skillet. Cook, stirring constantly, about 2 minutes. Remove from heat.

Preheat oven to 325°F. Spray 11- × 7-inch baking pan with nonstick cooking spray. Layer half of the eggplant slices in pan. Cover with lamb mixture. Top with remaining eggplant slices.

In small saucepan over low heat, melt margarine. Add remaining flour and cook, stirring constantly, about 1 minute. Gradually add milk and remaining pepper; cook, stirring constantly, 7 to 10 minutes or until thickened. Pour sauce over eggplant slices. Sprinkle with cheese. Bake 30 to 40 minutes or until hot and bubbly. MAKES 6 SERVINGS.

APPROXIMATE NUTRIENT ANALYSIS PER SERVING:

Calories □ 220
Protein □ 20 grams
Fat □ 8 grams
Carbohydrate □ 17 grams
Cholesterol □ 61 milligrams
Sodium □ 100 milligrams
Potassium □ 590 milligrams

% Calories from Fat □ 33
% Calories from Saturated Fat
  □ 16
% Calories from
  Monounsaturated Fat □ 14
% Calories from Polyunsaturated
  Fat □ 3
P/S □ 0.2

FOOD GROUP UNITS:

Vegetables □ 2
Grains □ ½
Meat and Alternatives:
  Moderately Low-Fat □ 2

Fat:
  Polyunsaturated □ 1

LAMB SHISH KABOBS

3 tablespoons fresh lemon
  juice
1 tablespoon olive oil
2 small garlic cloves, minced
¾ teaspoon dried oregano
⅛ teaspoon ground black
  pepper

1 pound boneless lamb, cut
  into 16 cubes
1 large green pepper, cut into
  16 squares (about 1½ cups)
2 onions, each cut into 8
  wedges (2 cups)
1 cup plain low-fat yogurt

□ In shallow dish, combine lemon juice, oil, garlic, oregano and pepper. Add lamb; toss well. Cover and refrigerate, stirring occasionally, about 1 hour.

Remove lamb from marinade, reserving marinade. Line broiler pan with foil. On each of four skewers, arrange 4 pieces of lamb, 4 green pepper squares and 4 onion wedges, then place on broiler pan. Broil 4 inches from heat, turning often and brushing with reserved marinade, 30 to 35 minutes. Transfer kabobs to serving platter.

Place yogurt in small bowl. Pour drippings from broiler pan into yogurt and mix well. Serve with kabobs. **MAKES 4 SERVINGS.**

APPROXIMATE NUTRIENT ANALYSIS PER SERVING:

Calories □ 265
Protein □ 27 grams
Fat □ 13 grams
Carbohydrate □ 10 grams
Cholesterol □ 93 milligrams
Sodium □ 105 milligrams
Potassium □ 575 milligrams

% Calories from Fat □ 43
% Calories from Saturated Fat
 □ 20
% Calories from
 Monounsaturated Fat □ 21
% Calories from Polyunsaturated
 Fat □ 2
P/S □ 0.1

FOOD GROUP UNITS:

Vegetables □ 2
Meat and Alternatives:
 Moderately Low-Fat □ 3
Milk Products:
 Moderately Low-Fat □ ¼

Fat:
 Monounsaturated □ ½

SAUERBRATEN STEW

1½ pounds beef stew meat
1 cup red wine vinegar
½ cup sliced onion
¾ cup water, divided
¼ cup dry red wine
1 bay leaf
2 whole cloves

½ teaspoon peppercorns
½ teaspoon salt
1 tablespoon vegetable oil
2 tablespoons all-purpose
 flour
6 gingersnaps, crushed
½ teaspoon sugar
3 cups cooked noodles
 (6 ounces dry)

□ Place beef in shallow dish. In medium bowl, combine vinegar, onion, ½ cup water, wine, bay leaf, cloves, peppercorns and salt; pour over beef and stir well. Cover and refrigerate, stirring occasionally, about 8 hours.

Remove beef from marinade, reserving marinade. Dry beef with paper towels. In large saucepan over medium-high heat, heat oil. Add beef and brown. Drain and discard excess fat. Add reserved marinade to saucepan; bring to a boil. Reduce heat, cover and simmer, stirring occasionally, 1½ to 2 hours or until beef is tender. With slotted spoon, remove beef. Strain liquid. Return liquid to saucepan with beef.

In small bowl, combine flour and ¼ cup water. Add to saucepan; cook 2 to 3 minutes or until thickened. Stir in gingersnap crumbs and sugar. Serve over noodles. **MAKES 6 SERVINGS.**

APPROXIMATE NUTRIENT ANALYSIS PER SERVING:

Calories □ 360
Protein □ 30 grams
Fat □ 14 grams
Carbohydrate □ 30 grams
Cholesterol □ 102 milligrams
Sodium □ 245 milligrams
Potassium □ 320 milligrams

% Calories from Fat □ 34
% Calories from Saturated Fat
□ 13
% Calories from
Monounsaturated Fat □ 15
% Calories from Polyunsaturated
Fat □ 16
P/S □ 0.4

FOOD GROUP UNITS:

Grains □ 2
Meat and Alternatives:
Moderately Low-Fat □ 3

Fat:
Polyunsaturated □ ½

CARAWAY PORK CHOPS

4 loin rib pork chops, cut ¾-inch thick
2 small potatoes, peeled and chopped (about 10 to 12 ounces)
½ cup chopped onion
1 can (16 ounces) tomatoes, chopped
½ teaspoon caraway seeds
⅛ teaspoon ground black pepper

□ Spray large nonstick skillet with nonstick cooking spray. In skillet over medium-high heat, brown pork chops. Remove from skillet. Add potatoes and onion to drippings in skillet; cook, stirring occasionally, about 5 minutes.

Return pork chops to skillet and add remaining ingredients; bring to a boil. Reduce heat, cover and simmer 45 minutes to 1 hour or until pork is tender. Transfer pork chops and vegetables to serving platter. Increase heat to high. Cook sauce until reduced slightly and thickened. Serve with pork. **MAKES 4 SERVINGS.**

APPROXIMATE NUTRIENT ANALYSIS PER SERVING:

Calories □ 260
Protein □ 21 grams
Fat □ 11 grams
Carbohydrate □ 20 grams
Cholesterol □ 63 milligrams
Sodium □ 235 milligrams
Potassium □ 785 milligrams

% Calories from Fat □ 37
% Calories from Saturated Fat □ 13
% Calories from Monounsaturated Fat □ 8
% Calories from Polyunsaturated Fat □ 6
P/S □ 0.4

FOOD GROUP UNITS:

Vegetables □ 1½
Grains □ ½
Meat and Alternatives:
 Moderately Low-Fat □ 3

Fat:
 Saturated □ ½

PORK AND APPLES

2 teaspoons vegetable oil
1 pound boneless pork
 shoulder, cut into ¾-inch
 cubes
½ cup sliced onion
1½ cups low-sodium beef
 broth
½ cup unsweetened apple
 juice
1 bay leaf

¼ teaspoon dried thyme
⅛ teaspoon ground black
 pepper
2 cups sliced celery
2 small apples, peeled, cored
 and sliced
1 tablespoon all-purpose flour
2 tablespoons water

□ In medium-size skillet over medium-high heat, heat oil. Add pork and brown. Remove from saucepan. Add onion to drippings in saucepan. Cook, stirring occasionally, 3 minutes or until soft. Return pork to saucepan. Add beef broth, apple juice, bay leaf, thyme and pepper; bring to a boil. Reduce heat, cover and simmer, stirring occasionally, about 1½ hours. Add celery; continue to simmer 30 minutes or until pork and celery are tender. Add apples; cook about 5 minutes.

In small bowl, combine flour and water. Add to saucepan. Cook, stirring frequently, 2 minutes or until thickened. Remove and discard bay leaf. MAKES 4 SERVINGS.

APPROXIMATE NUTRIENT ANALYSIS PER SERVING:

Calories □ 305
Protein □ 23 grams
Fat □ 15 grams
Carbohydrate □ 19 grams
Cholesterol □ 82 milligrams
Sodium □ 120 milligrams
Potassium □ 835 milligrams

% Calories from Fat □ 45
% Calories from Saturated Fat
 □ 15
% Calories from
 Monounsaturated Fat □ 19
% Calories from Polyunsaturated
 Fat □ 11
P/S □ 0.6

FOOD GROUP UNITS:

Vegetables □ 1
Fruits □ 1
Meat and Alternatives:
    Moderately Low-Fat □ 3

Fat:
    Polyunsaturated □ 1
    Saturated □ 1

VEGETABLES

SAUTÉED BROCCOLI

1 tablespoon + 1 teaspoon
    olive oil
2 large garlic cloves, coarsely
    chopped
4 cups fresh or 2 packages (10
    ounces each) frozen,
    thawed broccoli flowerets
⅓ cup low-sodium chicken
    broth

1 tablespoon fresh lemon
    juice
¼ teaspoon grated lemon peel
⅛ teaspoon ground black
    pepper

□ In large skillet over medium-high heat, heat oil. Add
garlic and cook, stirring constantly, about 30 seconds. Add
broccoli and cook, stirring occasionally, about 1 minute.

Add remaining ingredients. Reduce heat, cover and
simmer 5 to 7 minutes or until broccoli is tender-crisp.
MAKES 4 SERVINGS, about ⅔ cup each.

APPROXIMATE NUTRIENT ANALYSIS PER SERVING:

Calories □ 80
Carbohydrate □ 8 grams
Protein □ 5 grams
Fat □ 5 grams
Cholesterol □ 0
Sodium □ 40 milligrams
Potassium □ 305 milligrams

% Calories from Fat □ 45
% Calories from Saturated Fat
    □ 6
% Calories from
    Monounsaturated Fat □ 35
% Calories from Polyunsaturated
    Fat □ 4
P/S □ 0.6

SESAME GREEN BEANS

2 teaspoons vegetable oil
1 teaspoon sesame oil
¼ cup thinly sliced scallions
1 garlic clove, minced
1 package (9 ounces) frozen
    French-style green beans,
    thawed and well drained
    (1½ cups fresh)

¼ teaspoon ground ginger
⅛ teaspoon ground black
    pepper
⅔ cup fresh bean sprouts
1 tablespoon toasted sesame
    seeds
¼ teaspoon soy sauce

□ In large skillet over medium-high heat, heat vegetable and sesame oil. Add onion and garlic and cook, stirring frequently, about 3 minutes or until soft. Add beans, ginger and pepper and cook, stirring frequently, about 5 minutes. Stir in bean sprouts, sesame seeds and soy sauce and cook 1 minute or until heated through. MAKES 4 SERVINGS, about ½ cup each.

APPROXIMATE NUTRIENT ANALYSIS PER SERVING:

Calories □ 75
Protein □ 3 grams
Fat □ 5 grams
Carbohydrate □ 6 grams
Cholesterol □ 0
Sodium □ 30 milligrams
Potassium □ 170 milligrams

% Calories from Fat □ 56
% Calories from Saturated Fat
    □ 7
% Calories from
    Monounsaturated Fat □ 17
% Calories from Polyunsaturated
    Fat □ 32
P/S □ 3.9

BARBECUED POTATOES

1 pound unpeeled potatoes,
  washed (about 2 large)
1 tablespoon + 1 teaspoon
  margarine, melted
1 tablespoon honey

2 teaspoons chili powder
¼ teaspoon garlic powder
⅛ teaspoon ground black
  pepper

□ Preheat oven to 425°F. With knife, cut potatoes cross-wise into thin slices. Spray baking pan with nonstick cooking spray. Place potatoes on pan.

In small bowl, combine remaining ingredients until well blended; spread evenly over potatoes. Bake 15 to 20 minutes or until potatoes are fork-tender. MAKES 4 SERVINGS.

APPROXIMATE NUTRIENT ANALYSIS PER SERVING:

Calories □ 160
Protein □ 2 grams
Fat □ 4 grams
Carbohydrate □ 30 grams
Cholesterol □ 0
Sodium □ 70 milligrams
Potassium □ 475 milligrams

% Calories from Fat □ 23
% Calories from Saturated Fat
  □ 5
% Calories from
  Monounsaturated Fat □ 9
% Calories from Polyunsaturated
  Fat □ 9
P/S □ 2.1

FOOD GROUP UNITS:

Grains □ 1½

Fat:
  Polyunsaturated □ 1

Brussels Sprouts with Cream Sauce

2 cups frozen Brussels sprouts
1 tablespoon unsalted
   margarine
1 tablespoon chopped onion
1 garlic clove, minced
1 tablespoon all-purpose flour
½ cup skim milk
1 teaspoon dry white wine
⅛ teaspoon ground black
   pepper
1 tablespoon freshly grated
   Parmesan cheese

□ Cook Brussels sprouts according to package directions but without salt.

Meanwhile, in small saucepan over low heat, or in double boiler, melt margarine. Add onion and garlic and cook, stirring frequently, 3 minutes or until soft. Add flour and cook, stirring frequently, about 1 minute. Gradually add milk, wine and pepper and cook until thickened and smooth. Remove from heat; stir in cheese until melted. If sauce becomes too thick, add additional 1 to 2 tablespoons skim milk. Drain Brussels sprouts; pour sauce over sprouts. **MAKES 4 SERVINGS.**

APPROXIMATE NUTRIENT ANALYSIS PER SERVING:

Calories □ 85
Protein □ 5 grams
Fat □ 4 grams
Carbohydrate □ 10 grams
Cholesterol □ 2 milligrams
Sodium □ 65 milligrams
Potassium □ 315 milligrams

% Calories from Fat □ 36
% Calories from Saturated Fat
   □ 10
% Calories from
   Monounsaturated Fat □ 15
% Calories from Polyunsaturated
   Fat □ 11
P/S □ 1.2

Food Group Units:

Vegetables □ 1½

Fat:
   Polyunsaturated □ 1

SAUTÉED MIXED VEGETABLES

1 tablespoon unsalted
    margarine
1 teaspoon canola oil
1 cup sliced zucchini (1
    medium)
1 cup red pepper strips (½
    large)
½ cup sliced celery (2-3 small
    stalks)
¼ cup chopped onion

2 garlic cloves, minced
½ pound mushrooms,
    quartered (3 cups)
¾ teaspoon dried oregano
½ teaspoon dried basil
⅛ teaspoon crushed red
    pepper (optional)

□ In large nonstick skillet over medium-high heat, heat margarine and oil. Add zucchini, red pepper, celery, onion and garlic and cook, stirring frequently, 10 minutes or until tender-crisp. Add remaining ingredients and cook, stirring constantly, about 3 minutes. **MAKES 4 SERVINGS**, about ¾ cup each.

APPROXIMATE NUTRIENT ANALYSIS PER SERVING:

Calories □ 75
Protein □ 2 grams
Fat □ 5 grams
Carbohydrate □ 8 grams
Cholesterol □ 0
Sodium □ 20 milligrams
Potassium □ 455 milligrams

% Calories from Fat □ 50
% Calories from Saturated Fat
    □ 10
% Calories from
    Monounsaturated Fat □ 26
% Calories from Polyunsaturated
    Fat □ 14
P/S □ 2.1

FOOD GROUP UNITS:

Vegetables □ 2

Fat:
    Monounsaturated □ ½
    Polyunsaturated □ ½

RED CABBAGE AND APPLES

1 tablespoon unsalted
　margarine
¼ cup chopped onion
½ cup water
1 tablespoon white vinegar
¾ teaspoon caraway seeds

½ teaspoon sugar
⅛ teaspoon ground black
　pepper
2 cups shredded red cabbage
1 small apple, cored and
　sliced

□ In medium-size saucepan over medium-high heat, melt margarine. Add onion and cook, stirring frequently, 3 minutes or until soft. Add remaining ingredients, cover and simmer, stirring occasionally, 5 to 7 minutes or until cabbage is tender-crisp. MAKES 3 TO 4 SERVINGS, about ½ to 1 cup each.

APPROXIMATE NUTRIENT ANALYSIS PER SERVING:

Calories □ 85
Protein □ 1 gram
Fat □ 4 grams
Carbohydrate □ 12 grams
Cholesterol □ 0
Sodium □ 5 milligrams
Potassium □ 180 milligrams

% Calories from Fat □ 42
% Calories from Saturated Fat
　□ 8
% Calories from
　Monounsaturated Fat □ 19
% Calories from Polyunsaturated
　Fat □ 15
P/S □ 1.8

FOOD GROUP UNITS:

Vegetables □ ½
Fruits □ ½

Fat:
　Polyunsaturated □ 1

SNOW PEAS AND WATER CHESTNUTS

1 tablespoon + 1 teaspoon
   sesame oil
2 garlic cloves, minced
½ teaspoon finely chopped
   fresh ginger
1 package (6 ounces) frozen
   snow peas, thawed and well
   drained (1 ½ cups fresh)
⅓ cup sliced water chestnuts
½ cup coarsely chopped red
   pepper
1 teaspoon low-sodium soy
   sauce
⅛ teaspoon ground black
   pepper

□ In large nonstick skillet over medium-high heat, heat oil. Add garlic and ginger and cook about 1 minute. Add remaining ingredients and cook, stirring frequently, 5 to 7 minutes or until tender-crisp. MAKES 4 SERVINGS, about ½ cup each.

APPROXIMATE NUTRIENT ANALYSIS PER SERVING:

Calories □ 75
Protein □ 2 grams
Fat □ 5 grams
Carbohydrate □ 7 grams
Cholesterol □ 0
Sodium □ 55 milligrams
Potassium □ 170 milligrams

% Calories from Fat □ 54
% Calories from Saturated Fat
   □ 10
% Calories from
   Monounsaturated Fat □ 21.5
% Calories from Polyunsaturated
   Fat □ 22.5
P/S □ 3.0

FOOD GROUP UNITS:

Vegetables □ 2

Fat:
   Polyunsaturated □ 1

BROCCOLI AND CAULIFLOWER AU GRATIN

1 package (10 ounces) frozen, no-salt-added, or 2 cups fresh broccoli spears (7 to 9 spears)
1 package (10 ounces) frozen, no-salt-added, or 2 cups fresh cauliflower flowerets
1 cup skim milk
1 tablespoon cornstarch dissolved in 1 tablespoon cold water
1 tablespoon unsalted margarine, softened

¼ teaspoon dry mustard powder
¼ teaspoon ground black pepper
⅛ teaspoon ground nutmeg
⅛ teaspoon salt
1 cup grated low-fat Swiss or part-skim mozzarella cheese (about 3½ ounces)

□ Spray 1½- or 2-quart shallow baking dish with nonstick cooking spray. In medium-size saucepan, cook broccoli and cauliflower in small amount of unsalted, boiling water until almost tender. Drain and place in dish.

Preheat oven to 375°F. In small saucepan over medium heat, bring milk to a simmer. Add cornstarch mixture and cook, stirring constantly, until thickened, 1 to 2 minutes. Remove from heat and stir in margarine, mustard, pepper, nutmeg and salt. Pour over broccoli and cauliflower. Top with grated cheese. Bake, uncovered, 20 minutes or until bubbly. MAKES 6 SERVINGS.

APPROXIMATE NUTRIENT ANALYSIS PER SERVING:

Calories □ 120
Protein □ 9 grams
Fat □ 7 grams
Carbohydrate □ 8 grams
Cholesterol □ 1 milligram
Sodium □ 100 milligrams
Potassium □ 365 milligrams

% Calories from Fat □ 48
% Calories from Saturated Fat □ 25
% Calories from Monounsaturated Fat □ 14
% Calories from Polyunsaturated Fat □ 9
P/S □ 0.3

FOOD GROUP UNITS:

Vegetables □ 1½

Meat and Alternatives:
   Moderately Low-Fat □ ½

Fat:
   Polyunsaturated □ ½

CREAMED SPINACH

2 packages (10 ounces each)
   frozen, chopped, no-salt-
   added spinach
1 tablespoon unsalted
   margarine
¼ cup minced onion
2 garlic cloves, minced
1 tablespoon all-purpose flour

2 tablespoons sherry
¾ cup skim milk
1 tablespoon freshly grated
   Parmesan cheese
⅛ teaspoon ground black
   pepper
Dash ground nutmeg

□ Cook spinach according to package directions but without salt. Meanwhile, in medium-size saucepan over medium-high heat, melt margarine. Add onion and garlic and cook about 3 minutes. Stir in flour and cook, stirring, 1 minute. Stir in wine; cook about 30 seconds. Gradually add milk, stirring constantly. Continue cooking until thickened, about 2 to 3 minutes. Stir in Parmesan cheese, pepper and nutmeg. Drain spinach well and stir into sauce. **MAKES 6 SERVINGS.**

APPROXIMATE NUTRIENT ANALYSIS PER SERVING:

Calories □ 60
Protein □ 5 grams
Fat □ 3 grams
Carbohydrate □ 7 grams
Cholesterol □ 1 milligram
Sodium □ 110 milligrams
Potassium □ 605 milligrams

% Calories from Fat □ 35
% Calories from Saturated Fat
   □ 9
% Calories from
   Monounsaturated Fat □ 15
% Calories from Polyunsaturated
   Fat □ 11
P/S □ 1.2

FOOD GROUP UNITS:

Vegetables □ 1½   Fat:
                                  Polyunsaturated □ ½

BROILED TOMATO HALVES

3 large medium-ripe tomatoes   2 tablespoons chopped fresh
  (about 1¼ pounds)   parsley
2 tablespoons unsalted   ¼ teaspoon oregano
  margarine   ⅛ teaspoon garlic powder
¼ cup minced onion   ⅛ teaspoon ground black
1 cup fresh whole-wheat   pepper
  bread crumbs (2 slices)   2 teaspoons freshly grated
2 tablespoons oat bran   Parmesan cheese

□ Cut tomatoes in half crosswise; scoop out pulp. Chop pulp and place in small bowl; set aside. Place tomato halves in shallow baking dish and set aside.

Preheat oven to 400°F. In small skillet over medium heat, melt margarine. Add onion and cook 4 to 5 minutes or until tender. Add to chopped tomato pulp with bread crumbs, oat bran, parsley, oregano, garlic powder and pepper; blend well. Spoon mixture into reserved tomato halves. Sprinkle evenly with Parmesan cheese. Bake 12 minutes. Turn oven up to broil. Broil tomato halves 3 to 4 inches from heat source 1 to 2 minutes or until golden. **MAKES 6 SERVINGS.**

APPROXIMATE NUTRIENT ANALYSIS PER SERVING:

Calories □ 80   % Calories from Fat □ 49
Protein □ 2 grams   % Calories from Saturated Fat
Fat □ 5 grams   □ 11.5
Carbohydrate □ 9 grams   % Calories from
Cholesterol □ 1 milligram   Monounsaturated Fat □ 21.5
Sodium □ 75 milligrams   % Calories from Polyunsaturated
Potassium □ 185 milligrams   Fat □ 16
                                     P/S □ 1.4

Vegetables □ ½   Fat:
Grains □ ½   Polyunsaturated □ 1

GLAZED CARROTS

1 pound fresh carrots or 1 bag   ½ teaspoon grated lemon peel
  (16 ounces) frozen, no-salt-   ⅛ teaspoon ground black
  added baby carrots   pepper
2 tablespoons unsalted   ⅛ teaspoon cornstarch
  margarine   dissolved in 2 teaspoons
1 tablespoon brown sugar   cold water
⅓ cup unsweetened apple
  juice

□ If using fresh carrots, peel, cut into thirds crosswise then halve or quarter, depending on thickness. Cook in unsalted water until tender, 15 to 20 minutes; drain. If using frozen baby carrots, cook whole, according to package directions but without salt.

In large skillet over medium heat, melt margarine. Add carrots and brown sugar and toss to coat. Stir in apple juice, lemon peel and pepper. Bring to a simmer. Stir in cornstarch mixture. Cook, stirring, until thickened and clear, 1 to 2 minutes. **MAKES 4 SERVINGS.**

APPROXIMATE NUTRIENT ANALYSIS PER SERVING:

Calories □ 120   % Calories from Fat □ 42
Protein □ 1 gram   % Calories from Saturated Fat
Fat □ 6 grams   □ 8
Carbohydrate □ 17 grams   % Calories from
Cholesterol □ 0   Monounsaturated Fat □ 20
Sodium □ 40 milligrams   % Calories from Polyunsaturated
Potassium □ 405 milligrams   Fat □ 14
                                        P/S □ 1.7

Vegetables □ 1
Fruits □ ½

Fat:
  Polyunsaturated □ 1
Sugars □ ½

MASHED TURNIPS AND POTATOES

3 small potatoes, peeled and
  cubed (12 ounces)
1½ cups peeled, cubed
  turnips (about 8 ounces
  unpared)
1–2 tablespoons skim milk
2 tablespoons unsalted
  margarine

1 tablespoon chopped fresh
  parsley
1 tablespoon chopped chives
Dash ground red pepper
2 tablespoons freshly grated
  Parmesan cheese

□ In large saucepan over medium heat, cook potatoes and turnips in boiling water 20 to 30 minutes or until fork-tender; drain.

In large bowl, combine potatoes, turnips, milk and margarine; mash until fluffy. Stir in parsley, chives and red pepper. Spoon potato mixture into 1-quart shallow baking dish. Sprinkle with cheese. Broil 3 to 4 inches from heat 1 to 2 minutes or until lightly browned. MAKES 4 SERVINGS, about ½ cup each.

APPROXIMATE NUTRIENT ANALYSIS PER SERVING:

Calories □ 165
Protein □ 4 grams
Fat □ 7 grams
Carbohydrate □ 24 grams
Cholesterol □ 3 milligrams
Sodium □ 95 milligrams
Potassium □ 435 milligrams

% Calories from Fat □ 36
% Calories from Saturated Fat
  □ 10
% Calories from
  Monounsaturated Fat □ 15.5
% Calories from Polyunsaturated
  Fat □ 10.5
P/S □ 1.1

MUSHROOM STRUDEL

¼ cup + 1 tablespoon
  unsalted margarine, divided
½ cup chopped onion
1 garlic clove, minced
1½ pounds mushrooms,
  chopped (about 6 cups)
½ teaspoon dried thyme

⅛ teaspoon ground black
  pepper
2 tablespoons dry white wine
½ cup plain, dry, salt-free
  bread crumbs
1 egg white, slightly beaten
12 sheets phyllo leaves

□ In large nonstick skillet over medium-high heat, melt 1 tablespoon margarine. Add onion and garlic and cook, stirring occasionally, about 3 minutes. Add mushrooms, thyme and pepper and cook, stirring frequently, about 20 minutes. Add wine and cook, stirring frequently, 5 minutes or until all liquid has evaporated. Cool to room temperature; stir in bread crumbs and egg white.

Preheat oven to 375°F. Spray baking sheet with nonstick cooking spray. In small saucepan, melt remaining margarine. Place one phyllo sheet on damp towel. Brush lightly with margarine. Layer remaining phyllo sheets on top, brushing every other layer with margarine. Spoon mushroom mixture over dough, leaving 2-inch border on all sides. Fold shorter sides toward center. Roll up, starting from longer end. Place strudel seam-side-down on baking sheet. Brush with remaining margarine. Bake 20 to 30 minutes or until golden brown. Cool about 10 minutes on wire rack before slicing. MAKES 8 SERVINGS.

APPROXIMATE NUTRIENT ANALYSIS PER SERVING:

Calories □ 200
Protein □ 5 grams
Fat □ 10 grams
Carbohydrate □ 25 grams
Cholesterol □ 0
Sodium □ 150 milligrams
Potassium □ 370 milligrams

% Calories from Fat □ 42
% Calories from Saturated Fat
□ 11
% Calories from
Monounsaturated Fat □ 16
% Calories from Polyunsaturated
Fat □ 15
P/S □ 1.8

FOOD GROUP UNITS:

Vegetables □ 2
Grains □ 1½

Fat:
Polyunsaturated □ 1½

SALADS

MIXED VEGETABLE SALAD

2 cups broccoli flowerets (1
pound untrimmed)
½ pound mushrooms, sliced
(3 cups)
1 cup green pepper strips (1
medium)
1 cup red pepper strips (1
medium)
¼ cup chopped red onion
¼ cup vegetable oil

2 tablespoons red wine
vinegar
1 garlic clove, minced
¾ teaspoon dried basil
¼ teaspoon dried thyme
⅛ teaspoon ground black
pepper

□ In medium-size saucepan in 1 inch boiling water, bring broccoli to a boil. Reduce heat, cover and simmer 3 minutes or until tender-crisp; drain. Rinse under cold running water. Transfer to large bowl. Add mushrooms, green and red pepper and onion; toss.

In small bowl, combine oil, vineger, garlic, basil, thyme and pepper; pour over vegetables. Toss well. Cover and refrigerate about 2 hours. MAKES 6 SERVINGS, about 1 cup each.

APPROXIMATE NUTRIENT ANALYSIS PER SERVING:

Calories □ 110
Protein □ 2 grams
Fat □ 9 grams
Carbohydrate □ 6 grams
Cholesterol □ 0
Sodium □ 10 milligrams
Potassium □ 310 milligrams

% Calories from Fat □ 70
% Calories from Saturated Fat
□ 9
% Calories from
Monounsaturated Fat □ 17
% Calories from Polyunsaturated
Fat □ 44
P/S □ 4.6

FOOD GROUP UNITS:

Vegetables □ 1

Fat:
Polyunsaturated □ 2

WHEAT PILAF

2 tablespoons unsalted
  margarine
¾ cup sliced scallions
⅓ cup shredded carrots
¼ cup chopped green pepper
1 large garlic clove, minced

1 cup bulgur wheat
¼ cup chopped fresh parsley
2 cups boiling water
1 teaspoon grated lemon peel
⅛ teaspoon ground black
  pepper

□ In medium-size saucepan over medium-high heat, melt margarine. Add scallions, carrot, green pepper and garlic; cook 3 minutes. Stir in bulgur and parsley. Add water, lemon peel and black pepper. Reduce heat and simmer 20 minutes or until all liquid is absorbed. MAKES 6 SERVINGS, about ½ cup each.

APPROXIMATE NUTRIENT ANALYSIS PER SERVING:

Calories □ 150

Protein □ 3 grams

Fat □ 4 grams

Carbohydrates □ 26 grams

Cholesterol □ 0

Sodium □ 5 milligrams

Potassium □ 185 milligrams

% Calories from Fat □ 25

% Calories from Saturated Fat
□ 6

% Calories from
Monounsaturated Fat □ 11

% Calories from Polyunsaturated
Fat □ 8

P/S □ 1.7

FOOD GROUP UNITS:

Grains □ 1½

Vegetables □ ½

Fat:
Polyunsaturated □ 1

INDIAN RICE SALAD

⅔ cup brown rice

½ cup raisins

¼ cup slivered almonds,
toasted

¼ cup chopped celery

2 tablespoons chopped onion

3 tablespoons vegetable oil

2 tablespoons white vinegar

1 garlic clove, minced

1 teaspoon curry powder

½ teaspoon ground cumin

¼ teaspoon ground cinnamon

⅛ teaspoon ground black
pepper

□ Cook rice according to package directions but without salt. In medium-size bowl, combine rice, raisins, almonds, celery and onion; toss.

In small bowl, combine remaining ingredients; pour over salad. Toss well. Cover and refrigerate about 2 hours. MAKES 7 SERVINGS, about ½ cup each.

APPROXIMATE NUTRIENT ANALYSIS PER SERVING:

Calories □ 130

Protein □ 2 grams

Fat □ 8 grams

% Calories from Fat □ 55

% Calories from Saturated Fat
□ 7

Carbohydrate □ 14 grams
Cholesterol □ 0
Sodium □ 6 milligrams
Potassium □ 145 milligrams

% Calories from
Monounsaturated Fat □ 20
% Calories from Polyunsaturated
Fat □ 28
P/S □ 4.0

FOOD GROUP UNITS:

Fruits □ 1
Grains □ 2

Fat:
Polyunsaturated □ 2½

CREAMY CHICKEN SALAD

2 cups chopped cooked
chicken (1 pound 10
ounces raw, trimmed)
¾ cup 1-inch julienne
zucchini strips (1 small)
½ cup torn spinach leaves
¼ cup chopped carrots (1
small)
6 walnut halves, chopped
(2½ tablespoons)

¼ cup plain low-fat yogurt
2 tablespoons mayonnaise
1 small garlic clove, minced
¼ teaspoon dried tarragon
⅛ teaspoon ground black
pepper
Whole spinach leaves

□ In medium-size bowl, combine chicken, zucchini, spinach, carrots and walnuts; toss.

In small bowl, combine remaining ingredients; pour over salad. Toss well. Cover and refrigerate about 2 hours. Serve on whole spinach leaves. MAKES 4 SERVINGS, about ¾ cup each.

APPROXIMATE NUTRIENT ANALYSIS PER SERVING:

Calories □ 250
Protein □ 30 grams
Fat □ 12 grams
Carbohydrate □ 6 grams
Cholesterol □ 77 milligrams

% Calories from Fat □ 42
% Calories from Saturated Fat
□ 8
% Calories from
Monounsaturated Fat □ 13

Sodium □ 145 milligrams
Potassium □ 600 milligrams

% Calories from Polyunsaturated
Fat □ 21
P/S □ 2.7

FOOD GROUP UNITS:

Vegetables □ ½
Meat and Alternatives:
Very Low-Fat □ 3

Fat:
Polyunsaturated □ 2

TOFU SALAD

¼ cup vegetable oil
2 tablespoons red wine
vinegar
1 garlic clove, minced
½ teaspoon dried oregano
¼ teaspoon salt
⅛ teaspoon crushed red
pepper
8 ounces tofu (bean curd),
drained and cut into ½-inch
cubes (3½ cups)

2 cups chopped tomatoes
(about 2½ medium
tomatoes)
¼ pound mushrooms, sliced
(2 cups)
¼ cup sliced celery (1 large
stalk)
¼ cup chopped green pepper
¼ cup chopped fresh parsley
2 tablespoons chopped onion

□ In large bowl, combine oil, vinegar, garlic, oregano, salt and red pepper; mix well. Add tofu; toss. Cover and refrigerate, stirring occasionally, about 2 hours.

About 1 hour prior to serving, add vegetables; toss to coat. MAKES 6 SERVINGS, about ⅓ cup each.

APPROXIMATE NUTRIENT ANALYSIS PER SERVING:

Calories □ 130
Protein □ 4 grams
Fat □ 11 grams
Carbohydrate □ 6 grams
Cholesterol □ 0
Sodium □ 95 milligrams
Potassium □ 290 milligrams

% Calories from Fat □ 72
% Calories from Saturated Fat
□ 10
% Calories from
Monounsaturated Fat □ 18
% Calories from Polyunsaturated
Fat □ 44
P/S □ 4.6

PASTA AND VEGETABLE SALAD

4 ounces small shell macaroni
   (1¼ cups dry)
½ cup chopped broccoli
½ cup chopped carrots
¼ cup chopped red pepper
2 tablespoons chopped onion
¼ cup plain low-fat yogurt
1 tablespoon vegetable oil

2 teaspoons white vinegar
1 garlic clove, minced
1½ teaspoons dry mustard
   powder
⅛ teaspoon salt
⅛ teaspoon ground black
   pepper
Dash hot-pepper sauce
   (optional)

□ Cook pasta according to package directions but without salt.

Meanwhile, in medium-size saucepan in 1 inch boiling water, bring broccoli to a boil. Reduce heat, cover and simmer 2 minutes or until tender-crisp; drain. Rinse under cold running water.

In large bowl, combine drained pasta with broccoli, carrots, red pepper and onion; toss.

In small bowl, combine remaining ingredients; pour over salad. Toss well. Cover and refrigerate about 2 hours. **MAKES 4 SERVINGS**, about ¾ cup each.

APPROXIMATE NUTRIENT ANALYSIS PER SERVING:

Calories □ 125
Protein □ 4 grams
Fat □ 4 grams
Carbohydrate □ 19 grams
Cholesterol □ 1 milligram

% Calories from Fat □ 28
% Calories from Saturated Fat
   □ 5
% Calories from
   Monounsaturated Fat □ 7

Sodium □ 80 milligrams
Potassium □ 190 milligrams

% Calories from Polyunsaturated
Fat □ 16
P/S □ 3.5

FOOD GROUP UNITS:

Vegetables □ 2
Grains □ 1

Fat:
Polyunsaturated □ 1

WALDORF SALAD

2 small apples, cored and
chopped (1⅓ cups)
2 small pears, cored and
chopped (1½ cups)
1 small banana
½ avocado, sliced
½ cup chopped celery (2
medium stalks)

¼ cup raisins
12 walnut halves, chopped
(rounded ⅓ cup)
½ cup plain low-fat yogurt
1 tablespoon mayonnaise
1 teaspoon lemon juice

□ In medium bowl, combine all ingredients; toss well.
Cover and refrigerate about 2 hours. **MAKES 6 SERV-
INGS, about ¾ cup each.**

APPROXIMATE NUTRIENT ANALYSIS PER SERVING:

Calories □ 200
Protein □ 3 grams
Fat □ 10 grams
Carbohydrate □ 29 grams
Cholesterol □ 3 milligrams
Sodium □ 45 milligrams
Potassium □ 475 milligrams

% Calories from Fat □ 41
% Calories from Saturated Fat
□ 6.5
% Calories from
Monounsaturated Fat □ 16.5
% Calories from Polyunsaturated
Fat □ 18
P/S □ 2.9

FOOD GROUP UNITS:

Vegetables □ 1
Fruits □ 2 ½

Fat:
Polyunsaturated □ ½
Monounsaturated □ ½

RED POTATO SALAD

1 pound small red potatoes
   (about 8)
¾ cup cooked (about ⅓ cup
   dried) or canned, drained
   and rinsed white kidney
   beans
1 cup chopped red pepper (1
   large)
¾ cup sliced celery (3
   medium stalks)
¼ cup thinly sliced onion

¼ cup vegetable oil
2 tablespoons red wine
   vinegar
1 garlic clove, minced
¾ teaspoon dill weed
¼ teaspoon salt
⅛ teaspoon ground black
   pepper

□ In medium-size saucepan in 1 inch boiling water, bring potatoes to a boil. Reduce heat to low, cover and simmer 15 to 20 minutes or until fork-tender; drain. Cool to room temperature.

Cut potatoes into quarters; place in large bowl. Add beans, red pepper, celery and onion; toss.

In small bowl, combine remaining ingredients; pour over salad. Toss well. Cover and refrigerate about 2 hours. **MAKES 6 SERVINGS,** about ¾ to 1 cup each.

APPROXIMATE NUTRIENT ANALYSIS PER SERVING:

Calories □ 190
Protein □ 4 grams
Fat □ 9 grams
Carbohydrate □ 24 grams
Cholesterol □ 0
Sodium □ 100 milligrams
Potassium □ 500 milligrams

% Calories from Fat: □ 43
% Calories from Saturated Fat
   □ 6
% Calories from
   Monounsaturated Fat □ 10
% Calories from Polyunsaturated
   Fat □ 27
P/S □ 4.5

FOOD GROUP UNITS:

Grains □ 1

Fat:
   Polyunsaturated □ 1½

CONFETTI SLAW

1½ cups shredded green
   cabbage
½ cup shredded red cabbage
½ cup shredded carrots
2 tablespoons minced onion
2 tablespoons plain low-fat
   yogurt
2 tablespoons mayonnaise

1½ teaspoons skim milk
1½ teaspoons fresh lemon
   juice
¼ teaspoon celery seed
¼ teaspoon sugar
⅛ teaspoon ground black
   pepper

□ In large bowl, combine green and red cabbage, carrots
and onion; toss.

In small bowl, combine remaining ingredients; pour over
salad. Toss well. Cover and refrigerate about 2 hours.
MAKES 4 SERVINGS, about ¾ cup each.

APPROXIMATE NUTRIENT ANALYSIS PER SERVING:

Calories □ 75
Protein □ 1 gram
Fat □ 6 grams
Carbohydrate □ 5 grams
Cholesterol □ 5 milligrams
Sodium □ 60 milligrams
Potassium □ 180 milligrams

% Calories from Fat □ 66
% Calories from Saturated Fat
   □ 11
% Calories from
   Monounsaturated Fat □ 19
% Calories from Polyunsaturated
   Fat □ 36
P/S □ 3.3

FOOD GROUP UNITS:

Vegetables □ 1

Fat:
   Polyunsaturated □ 1

MOLDED SUNSHINE SALAD

1 can (11 ounces) mandarin
orange segments in light
syrup
2 cans (8 ounces each)
pineapple chunks in juice
1¼ cups orange juice
4½ teaspoons unflavored
gelatin
1 medium banana, sliced
(about 1 cup)

Water
1 teaspoon sugar
1 teaspoon grated lemon peel
½ cup plain nonfat yogurt
1 teaspoon vanilla extract

□ Drain mandarin orange segments, reserving syrup. Drain pineapple chunks, reserving juice. Place ¼ cup pineapple juice in small saucepan with reserved syrup and orange juice. Sprinkle 2½ teaspoons gelatin over juice mixture; let stand 5 minutes to soften gelatin. Cook over low heat until gelatin dissolves completely. Pour into shallow dish and refrigerate until syrupy, about 50 minutes. Stir in reserved mandarin orange segments and banana slices. Pour into 6-cup mold and refrigerate.

Meanwhile, pour remaining pineapple juice into measuring cup and add enough water to equal 1 cup. Place in small saucepan with sugar and lemon peel. Sprinkle with remaining 1½ teaspoons gelatin; let stand 5 minutes to soften gelatin. Cook over low heat until gelatin dissolves completely. Pour into shallow dish and refrigerate 15 minutes. Stir in yogurt, vanilla and reserved pineapple chunks (mixture will be very thin).

Gently spoon onto juice layer in mold. Juice layer should be almost firm. Cover and refrigerate until firm, several hours or overnight. Unmold onto serving platter. MAKES 12 SERVINGS, about ½ cup each.

APPROXIMATE NUTRIENT ANALYSIS PER SERVING:

Calories □ 70   % Calories from Fat □ 0
Protein □ 2 grams
Fat □ 0
Carbohydrate □ 16 grams
Cholesterol □ 1 milligram
Sodium □ 11 milligrams
Potassium □ 175 milligrams

FOOD GROUP UNITS:

Fruits □ 1   Sugars □ 1

SAUCES AND DRESSINGS

BARBECUE SAUCE

1 can (8 ounces) low-sodium   2 tablespoons minced onion
   tomato sauce   1½ tablespoons chili powder
1 tablespoon light brown   1 garlic clove, minced
   sugar   1 teaspoon dry mustard
2 tablespoons white vinegar

□ In small saucepan over medium heat, combine all ingredients and cook, stirring frequently, 15 to 20 minutes, or until slightly thickened. May be used as marinade or sauce. **MAKES 8 SERVINGS**, about 2 tablespoons each.

APPROXIMATE NUTRIENT ANALYSIS PER SERVING:

Calories □ 25   % Calories from Fat □ 0
Protein □ 1 gram
Fat □ 0

Carbohydrate □ 5 grams
Cholesterol □ 0
Sodium □ 25 milligrams
Potassium □ 40 milligrams

FOOD GROUP UNITS:

Vegetables □ 1

BASIC CREAM SAUCE

2 cups skim milk
2 tablespoons sherry
⅛ teaspoon ground black
   pepper

Dash ground nutmeg
2 tablespoons cornstarch
   dissolved in 2 tablespoons
   cold water

□ In medium-size saucepan over medium heat, bring milk, wine, pepper and nutmeg to a simmer, stirring occasionally to prevent scorching. Stir in cornstarch mixture and cook, stirring constantly, 3 to 4 minutes or until thickened and bubbly. MAKES 8 SERVINGS, about ¼ cup each.

VARIATIONS:

□ For salmon and fresh vegetables: add ¾ teaspoon dried dill weed, ½ teaspoon celery seed and ½ teaspoon dried tarragon.

□ For a Cajun-style sauce for veal, chicken or turkey: add ¼ teaspoon dried oregano, ⅛ teaspoon garlic powder, ⅛ teaspoon paprika and a few drops hot-pepper sauce.

□ For chicken, turkey or vegetables: add ½ teaspoon dried basil, ¼ teaspoon ground thyme and ⅛ teaspoon dry mustard.

□ For seafood and pasta: add 2 tablespoons chopped fresh parsley, 1 teaspoon grated lemon peel and ⅛ teaspoon garlic powder.

□ For vegetables, meats and beans: add 1 teaspoon dried savory.

APPROXIMATE NUTRIENT ANALYSIS PER SERVING:

Calories □ 30   % Calories from Fat □ 0
Protein □ 2 grams
Fat □ 0
Carbohydrate □ 5 grams
Cholesterol □ 1 milligram
Sodium □ 30 milligrams
Potassium □ 100 milligrams

FOOD GROUP UNITS:
Milk Products:
    Very Low-Fat □ ¼

Mushroom Sauce

2 tablespoons unsalted
  margarine
¼ pound mushrooms,
  quartered
2 tablespoons chopped onion
1 tablespoon all-purpose flour
1 cup low-sodium beef broth

¼ cup chopped fresh parsley
2 tablespoons Madeira wine
¼ teaspoon dried thyme
⅛ teaspoon ground black
  pepper

□ In medium-size saucepan over medium-high heat, melt margarine. Add mushrooms and onion and cook, stirring frequently, about 5 minutes. Add flour and cook, stirring constantly, about 1 minute. Gradually add remaining ingredients; bring to a boil. Cook mixture, stirring constantly, 3 to 4 minutes or until slightly thickened. May be used as a sauce for meats or vegetables. MAKES 10 SERVINGS, about 2 tablespoons each.

APPROXIMATE NUTRIENT ANALYSIS PER SERVING:

Calories □ 30
Protein □ 0
Fat □ 2 grams
Carbohydrate □ 2 grams
Cholesterol □ 0
Sodium □ 2 milligrams
Potassium □ 115 milligrams

% Calories from Fat □ 71
% Calories from Saturated Fat
  □ 14.5
% Calories from
  Monounsaturated Fat □ 33
% Calories from Polyunsaturated
  Fat □ 23.5
P/S □ 1.7

Food Group Units:

Vegetables □ ½

Fat:
  Polyunsaturated □ ½

CATSUP

1 tablespoon sugar
1½ tablespoons vinegar
1 can (6 ounces) tomato
    paste, canned without salt

2 teaspoons Worcestershire
    sauce
¼ teaspoon garlic powder
⅛ teaspoon ground black
    pepper

□ In small bowl, dissolve sugar in vinegar. Add remaining ingredients; blend well. Cover and refrigerate about 2 hours. MAKES 12 SERVINGS, about 1 tablespoon each.

APPROXIMATE NUTRIENT ANALYSIS PER SERVING:

Calories □ 15
Protein □ 1 gram
Fat □ 0
Carbohydrate □ 4 grams
Cholesterol □ 0
Sodium □ 15 milligrams
Potassium □ 140 milligrams

% Calories from Fat □ 0

FOOD GROUP UNITS:

Vegetables □ ½

CHUTNEY

1 cup peeled, finely chopped
    apples (2 small)
1 cup peeled, chopped pears
    (1½ medium)
½ cup raisins
½ cup firmly packed light
    brown sugar
½ cup cider vinegar

⅓ cup chopped onion
1 garlic clove, minced
¾ teaspoon ground cinnamon
½ teaspoon ground ginger
¼ teaspoon ground allspice
¼ teaspoon ground black
    pepper

□ In large saucepan, combine all ingredients; bring to a boil. Reduce heat and simmer, stirring occasionally, 40 minutes or until thickened. **MAKES 16 SERVINGS,** about 2 tablespoons each.

APPROXIMATE NUTRIENT ANALYSIS PER SERVING:

Calories □ 60
Protein □ 0
Fat □ 0
Carbohydrate □ 16 grams
Cholesterol □ 0
Sodium □ 3 milligrams
Potassium □ 115 milligrams

% Calories from Fat □ 0

FOOD GROUP UNITS:

Fruits □ 1

Sugars □ ½

SPICY TOMATO DRESSING

1⅓ cups low-sodium tomato
  or vegetable juice
¼ cup red wine vinegar
2 tablespoons olive oil
½ teaspoon dried oregano

¼ teaspoon dried thyme
⅛ teaspoon hot-pepper sauce
⅛ teaspoon garlic powder

□ In covered jar or shaker, combine all ingredients; refrigerate about 2 hours. Shake well before using. **MAKES 12 SERVINGS,** about 2 tablespoons each.

APPROXIMATE NUTRIENT ANALYSIS PER SERVING:

Calories □ 25
Protein □ 0
Fat □ 2 grams
Carbohydrate □ 2 grams
Cholesterol □ 0

% Calories from Fat □ 74
% Calories from Saturated Fat
  □ 10
% Calories from
  Monounsaturated Fat □ 59

Sodium □ 3 milligrams
Potassium □ 65 milligrams

% Calories from Polyunsaturated
Fat □ 5
P/S □ 0.6

FOOD GROUP UNITS:

Fat:
Monounsaturated □ ½

THOUSAND ISLAND DRESSING

1 cup plain low-fat yogurt
3 tablespoons mayonnaise
2 tablespoons low-sodium
chili sauce
1 tablespoon skim milk

1 tablespoon minced onion
1 tablespoon minced green
pepper
⅛ teaspoon garlic powder
⅛ teaspoon ground black
pepper

□ In small bowl, combine all ingredients; cover. Chill about 2 hours. Stir well before serving. **MAKES 12 SERV-INGS**, about 2 tablespoons each.

APPROXIMATE NUTRIENT ANALYSIS PER SERVING:

Calories □ 40
Protein □ 1 gram
Fat □ 3 grams
Carbohydrate □ 2 grams
Cholesterol □ 3 milligrams
Sodium □ 35 milligrams
Potassium □ 50 milligrams

% Calories from Fat □ 69
% Calories from Saturated Fat □
14
% Calories from
Monounsaturated Fat □ 20
% Calories from Polyunsaturated
Fat □ 35
P/S □ 2.4

FOOD GROUP UNITS:

Fat:
Polyunsaturated □ 1

CREAMY CUCUMBER DRESSING

¾ cup plain low-fat yogurt
⅓ cup peeled, seeded and
   minced cucumber (½
   medium)
3 tablespoons mayonnaise
1 tablespoon finely chopped
   green onion

1 tablespoon skim milk
1 teaspoon white vinegar
1 garlic clove, minced
⅛ teaspoon ground black
   pepper

□ In small bowl, combine all ingredients; mix well. Cover and refrigerate about 2 hours. Stir well before serving. **MAKES 12 SERVINGS,** about 2 tablespoons each.

APPROXIMATE NUTRIENT ANALYSIS PER SERVING:

Calories □ 35
Protein □ 1 gram
Fat □ 3 grams
Carbohydrate □ 2 grams
Cholesterol □ 3 milligrams
Sodium □ 30 milligrams
Potassium □ 60 milligrams

% Calories from Fat □ 72
% Calories from Saturated Fat
   □ 14
% Calories from
   Monounsaturated Fat □ 22
% Calories from Polyunsaturated
   Fat □ 36
P/S □ 2.6

FOOD GROUP UNITS:

Fat:
   Polyunsaturated □ 1

POPPY SEED DRESSING

¼ cup vegetable oil	1 teaspoon sugar
2 tablespoons white vinegar	½ teaspoon dried tarragon
1 tablespoon poppy seeds	⅛ teaspoon ground red pepper

□ In covered jar or shaker, combine all ingredients; refrigerate about 2 hours. Shake well before using. Serve over fruit or vegetable salads. MAKES 12 SERVINGS, about 2 teaspoons each.

APPROXIMATE NUTRIENT ANALYSIS PER SERVING:

Calories □ 45	% Calories from Fat □ 93
Protein □ 0	% Calories from Saturated Fat
Fat □ 5 grams	□ 12
Carbohydrate □ 1 gram	% Calories from
Cholesterol □ 0	Monounsaturated Fat □ 23.5
Sodium □ 0	% Calories from Polyunsaturated
Potassium □ 10 milligrams	Fat □ 57.5
	P/S □ 4.7

FOOD GROUP UNITS:

Fat:
  Polyunsaturated □ 1

ORANGE FRUIT DRESSING

1 cup plain low-fat yogurt	¼ teaspoon grated orange peel
2 tablespoons mayonnaise	¼ teaspoon ground cinnamon
2 tablespoons orange juice	⅛ teaspoon ground nutmeg
1 tablespoon honey	Dash ground red pepper

□ In small bowl, combine all ingredients. Cover and refrigerate about 2 hours. Stir well before serving. MAKES 10 SERVINGS, about 2 tablespoons each.

APPROXIMATE NUTRIENT ANALYSIS PER SERVING:

Calories □ 45
Protein □ 1 gram
Fat □ 3 grams
Carbohydrate □ 4 grams
Cholesterol □ 3 milligrams
Sodium □ 30 milligrams
Potassium □ 60 milligrams

% Calories from Fat □ 53
% Calories from Saturated Fat
 □ 12
% Calories from
 Monounsaturated Fat □ 15.5
% Calories from Polyunsaturated
 Fat □ 25.5
P/S □ 2.0

FOOD GROUP UNITS:

Fat:
 Polyunsaturated □ 1

BREADS

ZUCCHINI-CARROT BREAD

½ cup honey
¼ cup canola oil
1 large egg
1½ teaspoons vanilla extract
¾ cup all-purpose flour
½ cup whole-wheat flour
½ cup oat bran

1½ teaspoons baking powder
1½ teaspoons ground
 cinnamon
⅛ teaspoon salt
1 cup shredded zucchini
1 cup shredded carrots
2 teaspoons grated orange
 peel
¼ cup walnuts, chopped
 (optional)

□ Preheat oven to 350°F. Spray 8- × 5-inch loaf pan with nonstick cooking spray. In large bowl, whisk together honey, oil, egg and vanilla. In another bowl, stir together the flours, oat bran, baking powder, cinnamon and salt. Add dry ingredients to honey mixture with zucchini, carrots and orange peel. Stir to blend well. Add walnuts (if desired). Spoon into pan. Bake 50 to 60 minutes or until toothpick inserted in center comes out clean. Cool completely on wire rack. MAKES 16 SERVINGS, each a ½-inch slice.

APPROXIMATE NUTRIENT ANALYSIS PER SERVING:

Calories □ 125
Protein □ 2 grams
Fat □ 5 grams
Carbohydrate □ 19 grams
Cholesterol □ 17 milligrams
Sodium □ 55 milligrams
Potassium □ 100 milligrams

% Calories from Fat □ 35
% Calories from Saturated Fat
   □ 4
% Calories from
   Monounsaturated Fat □ 18
% Calories from Polyunsaturated
   Fat □ 13
P/S □ 3.7

FOOD GROUP UNITS:

Grains □ 1

Fat:
   Monounsaturated □ 1
Sugars □ 1

HONEY BRAN MUFFINS

1½ cups oat bran, divided
½ cup boiling water
½ cup all-purpose flour
½ cup whole-wheat flour
1½ teaspoons baking soda
⅛ teaspoon salt

1 cup no-salt-added
   buttermilk
¼ cup honey
2½ tablespoons vegetable oil
1 egg
½ cup raisins (optional)*

□ Preheat oven to 400°F. Spray muffin tin with nonstick cooking spray. In large bowl, stir together ½ cup bran and

*Fresh blueberries (⅔ cup) may be substituted for raisins.

water; let stand about 5 minutes. In small bowl, combine remaining bran with all-purpose and whole-wheat flour, baking soda and salt.

In another small bowl, combine buttermilk, honey, oil and egg. Add dry and wet ingredients to wet bran; stir just until moistened. Fold in raisins. Pour batter into muffin tin. Bake 20 minutes or until toothpick inserted in center of muffin comes out clean. **MAKES 12 MUFFINS.**

APPROXIMATE NUTRIENT ANALYSIS PER SERVING:

Calories ◻ 145
Protein ◻ 5 grams
Fat ◻ 4 grams
Carbohydrate ◻ 27 grams
Cholesterol ◻ 24 milligrams
Sodium ◻ 145 milligrams
Potassium ◻ 138 milligrams

% Calories from Fat ◻ 23
% Calories from Saturated Fat
  ◻ 4
% Calories from
  Monounsaturated Fat ◻ 7
% Calories from Polyunsaturated
  Fat ◻ 12
P/S ◻ 3.2

FOOD GROUP UNITS:

Grains ◻ 1½

Fat:
  Polyunsaturated ◻ 1
Sugars ◻ ½

CRACKED WHEAT BREAD

⅓ cup skim milk, scalded
⅓ cup molasses
3 tablespoons unsalted
  margarine
1 teaspoon salt
1⅓ cups warm water (105–
  115°F)
1 package active dry yeast

4–4½ cups all-purpose flour,
  divided
¾ cup whole-wheat flour
⅔ cup cracked wheat (bulgur)
1 egg white
1 tablespoon water

□ In small bowl, combine milk, molasses, margarine and salt. In large bowl, sprinkle yeast over warm water; set aside 5 minutes or until yeast dissolves. With whisk, beat in milk mixture. Stir in 3 cups all-purpose flour, whole-wheat flour and cracked wheat until smooth. Mix in enough additional flour to make a soft dough.

Turn dough onto lightly floured surface; knead 10 minutes or until smooth and elastic, adding more flour as needed. Place dough in large greased bowl, turning to expose greased portion. Cover with towel; set aside in warm place to rise 1½ hours or until doubled.

Punch down dough. Spray 9- × 5-inch loaf pan with nonstick cooking spray. With lightly floured rolling pin, roll dough into 12- × 8-inch rectangle. Starting with narrow edge, roll dough; seal edges. Place seam-side-down in pan. Cover with towel; set aside in warm place to rise 1 hour or until doubled.

Meanwhile, preheat oven to 375°F. In small bowl, combine egg white and water; beat slightly. Brush over surface of dough. Bake 50 minutes or until golden brown. Remove from pan and cool on wire rack. MAKES 18 SERVINGS.

APPROXIMATE NUTRIENT ANALYSIS PER SERVING:

Calories □ 75
Protein □ 2 grams
Fat □ 2 grams
Carbohydrate □ 13 grams
Cholesterol □ 0
Sodium □ 115 milligrams
Potassium □ 105 milligrams

% Calories from Fat □ 24
% Calories from Saturated Fat
□ 5
% Calories from
Monounsaturated Fat □ 11
% Calories from Polyunsaturated
Fat □ 8
P/S □ 1.6

FOOD GROUP UNITS:

Grains □ 1

Fat:
Polyunsaturated □ ½

POTATO ROLLS

⅓ cup skim milk, scalded
2 tablespoons sugar
2 tablespoons margarine
½ teaspoon salt
⅛ teaspoon ground black
   pepper

1 teaspoon active dry yeast
⅓ cup warm water (105–
   115°F)
½ cup mashed potato (1 small
   potato)
2–2½ cups all-purpose flour

□ In small bowl, combine milk, sugar, margarine, salt and pepper; cool to lukewarm.

In large bowl, sprinkle yeast over warm water; set aside 5 minutes or until yeast dissolves. With whisk, beat milk mixture into mashed potato until smooth. Stir in 1½ cups flour until smooth. Add enough additional flour to make a soft dough.

Turn dough onto a lightly floured surface; knead 10 minutes or until smooth and elastic, adding more flour as needed. Place dough in greased bowl, turning to expose greased portion. Cover with towel; set aside in warm place to rise 1 hour or until doubled.

Spray muffin tin with nonstick cooking spray. Punch down dough; divide into 12 pieces. Shape into 2-inch balls. With scissors, cut each ball in half, then into quarters, cutting through almost to bottom of rolls. Place each cut potato roll in muffin tin. Cover with towel; set aside in warm place to rise 45 minutes or until doubled.

Meanwhile, preheat oven to 400°F. Bake rolls 15 to 20 minutes or until golden brown. MAKES 6 SERVINGS, 2 rolls each.

APPROXIMATE NUTRIENT ANALYSIS PER SERVING:

Calories □ 265
Protein □ 6 grams
Fat □ 4 grams

% Calories from Fat □ 15
% Calories from Saturated Fat
   □ 3.5

Carbohydrate □ 49 grams
Cholesterol □ 0
Sodium □ 225 milligrams
Potassium □ 155 milligrams

% Calories from
Monounsaturated Fat □ 6
% Calories from Polyunsaturated
Fat □ 5.5
P/S □ 1.9

FOOD GROUP UNITS:

Vegetables □ 1
Grains □ 2½

Fat:
Polyunsaturated □ 1

PRUNE AND NUT BREAD

2 cups all-purpose flour
1 cup whole-wheat flour
⅓ cup sugar
1 tablespoon + 1 teaspoon
baking powder
¼ teaspoon salt
1 ½ cups skim milk

1 egg
3 tablespoons unsalted
margarine, melted
1 teaspoon vanilla extract
36 pitted prunes, chopped
(3 cups chopped)
30 whole shelled almonds,
chopped

□ Preheat oven to 325° F. Spray 9- × 5-inch loaf pan with nonstick cooking spray. In large bowl, combine all-purpose and whole-wheat flour, sugar, baking powder and salt; set aside.

In small bowl, combine milk, egg, margarine and vanilla; with fork, beat slightly. Stir in flour mixture until moistened. Gently fold in prunes and almonds; spoon into pan. Bake 45 to 60 minutes or until toothpick inserted in center comes out clean. Cool in pan about 10 minutes. Remove from pan; cool on wire rack. MAKES 18 SERVINGS.

APPROXIMATE NUTRIENT ANALYSIS PER SERVING:

Calories □ 200
Protein □ 4 grams
Fat □ 3 grams

% Calories from Fat □ 15
% Calories from Saturated Fat
□ 3

Carbohydrate □ 41 grams
Cholesterol □ 16 milligrams
Sodium □ 120 milligrams
Potassium □ 295 milligrams

% Calories from
  Monounsaturated Fat □ 7
% Calories from Polyunsaturated
  Fat □ 5
P/S □ 1.4

FOOD GROUP UNITS:

Fruits □ 1
Grains □ 1½

Fat:
  Polyunsaturated □ 1

GINGERBREAD

1 cup all-purpose flour
½ teaspoon baking soda
⅛ teaspoon salt
½ teaspoon ground ginger
¼ teaspoon ground cinnamon
⅛ teaspoon ground cloves

⅛ teaspoon ground allspice
3 tablespoons vegetable
  shortening
2 tablespoons sugar
¼ cup molasses
¼ cup boiling water

□ Preheat oven to 350° F. Spray 8- × 4-inch loaf pan with nonstick cooking spray. In medium bowl, combine flour, baking soda, salt and spices; set aside.

In large bowl with mixer at medium speed, cream shortening and sugar until light and fluffy; beat in molasses and boiling water. Stir in dry ingredients until moistened. Pour batter into pan. Bake 30 to 35 minutes or until toothpick inserted in center comes out clean. Cool in pan on wire rack about 10 minutes. Remove from pan and cool completely on rack. MAKES 16 SERVINGS.

APPROXIMATE NUTRIENT ANALYSIS PER SERVING:

Calories □ 70
Protein □ 1 gram
Fat □ 2 grams
Carbohydrate □ 11 grams
Cholesterol □ 0

% Calories from Fat □ 32
% Calories from Saturated Fat
  □ 9
% Calories from
  Monounsaturated Fat □ 14

Sodium □ 40 milligrams
Potassium □ 55 milligrams

% Calories from Polyunsaturated
  Fat □ 9
P/S □ 1.0

FOOD GROUP UNITS:

Grains □ ½

Fat:
  Monounsaturated □ ½

DESSERTS

OATMEAL APPLESAUCE COOKIES

1 cup all-purpose flour
¼ cup quick-cooking oats,
  uncooked
¾ teaspoon baking soda
¼ teaspoon ground cinnamon
Dash ground cloves

2 tablespoons margarine
¼ cup sugar
1 egg, slightly beaten
½ cup unsweetened
  applesauce

□ Preheat oven to 375°F. Spray baking sheets with nonstick cooking spray. In large bowl, combine flour, oats, baking soda, cinnamon and cloves; set aside.

With mixer at low speed, cream margarine and sugar until light and fluffy; beat in egg and applesauce. Stir in dry ingredients until smooth. Drop cookie batter onto baking sheets by teaspoonsful. Bake 6 to 8 minutes or until browned. Cool on wire racks. MAKES 8 SERVINGS, 3 cookies each.

APPROXIMATE NUTRIENT ANALYSIS PER SERVING:

Calories □ 125
Protein □ 3 grams
Fat □ 4 grams
Carbohydrate □ 21 grams
Cholesterol □ 34 milligrams

% Calories from Fat □ 27
% Calories from Saturated Fat
  □ 6
% Calories from
  Monounsaturated Fat □ 11

Sodium □ 125 milligrams
Potassium □ 40 milligrams

% Calories from Polyunsaturated
 Fat □ 10
P/S □ 1.6

FOOD GROUP UNITS:

Grains □ 1

Fat:
 Polyunsaturated □ 1
Sugars □ ½

MOCHA MERINGUES

1 egg white, at room
 temperature
⅛ teaspoon cream of tartar
2 tablespoons sugar

¼ teaspoon vanilla extract
1 tablespoon unsweetened
 cocoa powder
½ teaspoon instant coffee
 powder

□ Preheat oven to 250°F. Line baking sheets with foil. In medium bowl with mixer at high speed, beat egg white and cream of tartar until soft peaks form; gradually add sugar and vanilla. Gently fold in cocoa and coffee powder. Drop meringue onto baking sheets by teaspoonful 2 inches apart. Bake 40 minutes or until firm. Turn off oven. Let cookies cool in oven 1 hour without opening door. MAKES 4 SERVINGS, 3 cookies each.

APPROXIMATE NUTRIENT ANALYSIS PER SERVING:

Calories □ 30
Protein □ 1 gram
Fat □ 0
Carbohydrate □ 7 grams
Cholesterol □ 0
Sodium □ 15 milligrams
Potassium □ 40 milligrams

% Calories from Fat □ 0

FOOD GROUP UNITS:

Sugars □ ½

APPLE CRISP

3 large baking apples (such as Rome Beauty), peeled, cored, and sliced (about 1½ pounds)
2 tablespoons fresh lemon juice
¼ teaspoon grated lemon peel
¼ cup whole-wheat flour

¼ cup oat bran
2 tablespoons light brown sugar
1 teaspoon ground cinnamon
¼ teaspoon ground allspice
¼ cup margarine, softened

□ Preheat oven to 350°F. Spray 8-inch square baking pan with nonstick cooking spray. Arrange apples in pan. Sprinkle with lemon juice and lemon peel.

In small bowl, combine flour, bran, brown sugar, cinnamon and allspice. Cut in margarine with pastry blender until mixture resembles coarse crumbs. Sprinkle over apples. Bake 30 to 40 minutes until lightly browned. MAKES 6 SERVINGS.

APPROXIMATE NUTRIENT ANALYSIS PER SERVING:

Calories □ 180
Protein □ 2 grams
Fat □ 8 grams
Carbohydrate □ 29 grams
Cholesterol □ 0
Sodium □ 105 milligrams
Potassium □ 200 milligrams

% Calories from Fat □ 38
% Calories from Saturated Fat □ 7
% Calories from Monounsaturated Fat □ 15
% Calories from Polyunsaturated Fat □ 16
P/S □ 2.1

FOOD GROUP UNITS:

Fruits □ 2
Grains □ ½

Fat:
Polyunsaturated □ 1

ORANGE SORBET

2 cups orange juice
2 tablespoons fresh lemon
    juice
2 tablespoons sugar

½ teaspoon grated orange
    peel
1 egg white

□ In small saucepan over low heat, combine orange juice, lemon juice, sugar and orange peel; cook until sugar dissolves. Pour into large bowl; cool to room temperature.

In medium bowl with mixer at high speed, beat egg white until stiff peaks form; gently fold into orange juice. Pour mixture into a shallow metal pan. Freeze 2 hours or until partially frozen.

Spoon mixture into medium bowl. With mixer, beat until smooth. Freeze 3 hours or until solid. Let stand at room temperature about 10 minutes prior to serving. **MAKES 4 SERVINGS.**

APPROXIMATE NUTRIENT ANALYSIS PER SERVING:

Calories □ 85
Protein □ 2 grams
Fat □ 0
Carbohydrate □ 20 grams
Cholesterol □ 0
Sodium □ 15 milligrams
Potassium □ 260 milligrams

% Calories from Fat □ 0

FOOD GROUP UNITS:

Fruits □ 1
Meat and Alternatives:
    Very Low-Fat □ ¼

Sugars □ ½

BAKED BANANAS

2 small bananas, cut in half
   lengthwise
¼ cup raisins
2 tablespoons margarine,
   melted
1 tablespoon light brown
   sugar

½ teaspoon ground allspice
¼ teaspoon ground cinnamon
Dash ground nutmeg

□ Preheat oven to 450°F. Arrange bananas in 9-inch pie plate; sprinkle with raisins. In small bowl, combine remaining ingredients; pour over bananas. Bake 10 to 15 minutes or until hot and bubbly. **MAKES 4 SERVINGS.**

APPROXIMATE NUTRIENT ANALYSIS PER SERVING:

Calories □ 145
Protein □ 1 gram
Fat □ 6 grams
Carbohydrate □ 25 grams
Cholesterol □ 0
Sodium □ 80 milligrams
Potassium □ 320 milligrams

% Calories from Fat □ 35
% Calories from Saturated Fat
   □ 7
% Calories from
   Monounsaturated Fat □ 14
% Calories from Polyunsaturated
   Fat □ 14
P/S □ 2.0

FOOD GROUP UNITS:

Fruits □ 2

Fat:
   Polyunsaturated □ 1

CHERRY COBBLER

1 can (16 ounces) cherries in
juice
2 tablespoons quick-cooking
tapioca
2 tablespoons light brown
sugar
¼ teaspoon ground cinnamon
Dash ground cloves

½ cup all-purpose flour
¾ teaspoon baking powder
⅛ teaspoon salt
2 tablespoons margarine
¼ cup skim milk

□ Preheat oven to 375°F. In small saucepan, combine cherries and their juice, tapioca, brown sugar, cinnamon and cloves; let stand about 15 minutes. Over low heat, cook, stirring occasionally, 15 minutes or until slightly thickened. Pour mixture into 9-inch pie plate.

In small bowl, combine flour, baking powder and salt; mix well. With pastry blender, cut in margarine until mixture crumbles; stir in milk. Drop dough in four mounds over cherries. Bake 30 minutes or until lightly browned. **MAKES 6 SERVINGS.**

APPROXIMATE NUTRIENT ANALYSIS PER SERVING:

Calories □ 145
Protein □ 2 grams
Fat □ 4 grams
Carbohydrate □ 26 grams
Cholesterol □ 0
Sodium □ 145 milligrams
Potassium □ 145 milligrams

% Calories from Fat □ 24
% Calories from Saturated Fat
□ 5
% Calories from
Monounsaturated Fat □ 9.5
% Calories from Polyunsaturated
Fat □ 9.5
P/S □ 2.1

FOOD GROUP UNITS:

Fruits □ 1½
Grains □ 1½

Fat:
Polyunsaturated □ 1
Sugars □ ⅓

FRUIT PARFAITS

2 medium pears, cored and
  coarsely chopped (1½
  cups)
2 medium oranges, peeled,
  sectioned and cut into bite-
  size pieces (1¾ cups)
1 medium banana, sliced
  (1 cup)
1 cup strawberries, sliced

1½ cups raspberries
¾ cup orange juice
½ teaspoon vanilla extract
2 tablespoons creme de cassis
  (optional)

□ In large bowl, combine fruits. In small bowl, combine
remaining ingredients; pour over fruits and mix well. Cover
and refrigerate, stirring occasionally, about 2 hours. Spoon
into parfait glasses with marinade. **MAKES 6 SERVINGS.**

APPROXIMATE NUTRIENT ANALYSIS PER SERVING:

Calories □ 130
Protein □ 2 grams
Fat □ 1 gram
Carbohydrate □ 30 grams
Cholesterol □ 0
Sodium □ 2 milligrams
Potassium □ 405 milligrams

% Calories from Fat □ 5
% Calories from Saturated Fat
  □ 1
% Calories from
  Monounsaturated Fat □ 1.5
% Calories from Polyunsaturated
  Fat □ 2.5
P/S □ 3.6

FOOD GROUP UNITS:

Fruits □ 2

CARROT SPICE CAKE

½ cup apple juice
½ cup honey
½ cup water
1 cup shredded carrots
⅓ cup raisins
2 tablespoons unsalted
  margarine
1 teaspoon ground cinnamon
1 teaspoon ground allspice
¼ teaspoon ground nutmeg

⅛ teaspoon ground cloves
1 cup all-purpose flour
¾ cup whole-wheat flour
1 teaspoon baking powder
1 teaspoon baking soda
⅛ teaspoon salt
1 large egg
1–2 tablespoons
  confectioners' sugar

□ In medium-size saucepan, combine apple juice, honey, water, carrots, raisins, margarine and spices. Over medium-high heat, bring to a boil. Reduce heat, cover and simmer 10 minutes. Remove from heat and allow to cool (about 1 hour), stirring occasionally to release steam.

Meanwhile, in large bowl, stir together the flours, baking powder, baking soda and salt.

Preheat oven to 375°F. Spray 8-inch square baking pan with nonstick cooking spray. When carrot mixture is cool, whisk in egg. Pour into flour mixture and stir until well blended. Pour into pan. Bake 25 to 30 minutes or until toothpick inserted in center comes out clean. Cool on wire rack 10 minutes. Remove from pan and cool completely. Dust with confectioners' sugar. MAKES 16 SERVINGS.

APPROXIMATE NUTRIENT ANALYSIS PER SERVING:

Calories □ 115
Protein □ 2 grams
Fat □ 2 grams
Carbohydrate □ 24 grams
Cholesterol □ 17 milligrams
Sodium □ 95 milligrams
Potassium □ 95 milligrams

% Calories from Fat □ 15
% Calories from Saturated Fat
  □ 3
% Calories from
  Monounsaturated Fat □ 7
% Calories from Polyunsaturated
  Fat □ 5
P/S □ 1.2

FOOD GROUP UNITS:

Grains □ 1

Fruits □ ½

Fat:

Polyunsaturated □ ½

Sugars □ ½

PEARS WITH CHOCOLATE MINT SAUCE

1½ cups water

½ cup dry white wine

6 small pears, pared and
cored (about 2¼ pounds)

2 tablespoons unsweetened
cocoa powder

2 tablespoons water

1 tablespoon sugar

2½ teaspoons cornstarch

1 cup evaporated skim milk

⅛ teaspoon mint extract

□ In large saucepan, bring water and wine to a boil; add pears. Cover and simmer 30 to 40 minutes or until tender.

Meanwhile, in small saucepan, mix cocoa, water, sugar and cornstarch; stir in milk. Over low heat, cook, stirring constantly, until thickened. Remove from heat; add mint extract. Cover and refrigerate about 2 hours. Transfer pears to serving plate. Serve with sauce. **MAKES 6 SERVINGS.**

APPROXIMATE NUTRIENT ANALYSIS PER SERVING:

Calories □ 150

Protein □ 4 grams

Fat □ 1 gram

Carbohydrate □ 34 grams

Cholesterol □ 0

Sodium □ 50 milligrams

Potassium □ 395 milligrams

% Calories from Fat □ 5

% Calories from Saturated Fat
□ 1.7

% Calories from
Monounsaturated Fat □ 2

% Calories from Polyunsaturated
Fat □ 1.3

P/S □ 0.7

FOOD GROUP UNITS:

Fruits □ 1
Grains □ 1½
Milk Products:
  Very Low-Fat □ ¼

STRAWBERRY CHIFFON DESSERT

1½ cups fresh or frozen,
  thawed unsweetened
  strawberries
1 envelope unflavored gelatin
½ cup cold water
½ cup orange juice

2 tablespoons sugar
1 tablespoon rum
1 teaspoon vanilla extract
2 egg whites

□ In blender or food processor, puree strawberries; set aside.

In small saucepan, sprinkle gelatin over cold water; set aside 5 minutes or until gelatin softens. Over low heat, cook, stirring constantly, 5 minutes or until gelatin dissolves; pour into large bowl. Cool about 5 minutes; beat in orange juice, sugar, rum, vanilla and pureed strawberries. Cover and refrigerate 1 hour or until mixture mounds slightly when dropped from a spoon.

In medium bowl with mixer at high speed, beat egg whites until stiff peaks form. Gently fold into gelatin mixture; spoon into parfait glasses. Refrigerate until firm. MAKES 4 SERVINGS.

APPROXIMATE NUTRIENT ANALYSIS PER SERVING:

Calories □ 80
Protein □ 4 grams
Fat □ 0
Carbohydrate □ 14 grams
Cholesterol □ 0

% Calories from Fat □ 0

Sodium □ 30 milligrams
Potassium □ 220 milligrams

FOOD GROUP UNITS:

Fruits □ 1   Sugars □ ½
Meat and Alternatives:
   Very Low-Fat □ ½

CHOCO-BANANA CREAM PUFFS

¾ cup water, divided   2 tablespoons unsweetened
2 tablespoons margarine   cocoa powder
½ cup all-purpose flour   2 tablespoons sugar
2 eggs   1 cup plain low-fat yogurt
2 teaspoons unflavored gelatin   ½ teaspoon vanilla extract
1 small banana, mashed   ⅛ teaspoon ground cinnamon

□ Preheat oven to 375°F. Spray baking sheet with non-stick cooking spray. In small saucepan over high heat, bring ½ cup water and margarine to a boil; reduce heat to low. With wooden spoon, vigorously stir in flour until mixture forms ball and leaves side of pan; remove from heat. Add eggs, one at a time, beating well after each addition. Drop batter onto baking sheet in 6 large mounds about 3 inches apart. Bake 30 minutes or until puffy and golden brown. Cut off tops and reserve. Remove and discard soft dough in center. Cool on wire racks.

Meanwhile, in small saucepan, sprinkle gelatin over remaining ¼ cup cold water; set aside 5 minutes or until gelatin softens. Over low heat, cook, stirring constantly, 5 minutes or until gelatin dissolves; pour into medium bowl and cool 3 minutes. Beat in banana, cocoa and sugar until smooth. Stir in yogurt, vanilla and cinnamon. Cover and refrigerate. Spoon an equal amount of mixture into each cream puff. Cover with tops. MAKES 6 SERVINGS.

APPROXIMATE NUTRIENT ANALYSIS PER SERVING:

Calories □ 165
Protein □ 6 grams
Fat □ 7 grams
Carbohydrate □ 21 grams
Cholesterol □ 94 milligrams
Sodium □ 100 milligrams
Potassium □ 230 milligrams

% Calories from Fat □ 36
% Calories from Saturated Fat
  □ 11
% Calories from
  Monounsaturated Fat □ 15
% Calories from Polyunsaturated
  Fat □ 10
P/S □ 1.1

FOOD GROUP UNITS:

Grains □ 1
Meat and Alternatives:
  Very Low-Fat □ ½

Fat:
  Polyunsaturated □ 1
Sugars □ ½

PEACH YOGURT PIE

16 graham crackers (each 2½-
  inches square), crushed
  (about 1 cup)
¼ cup bran flake, crushed
3 tablespoons + 1 teaspoon
  margarine, melted
¼ teaspoon ground cinnamon
1 envelope unflavored gelatin
⅔ cup unsweetened apple
  juice

1 package (20 ounces) frozen,
  unsweetened peaches,
  thawed and drained (about
  3 cups), divided
1½ cups plain low-fat yogurt
¼ cup sugar
1 teaspoon vanilla extract
¼ teaspoon ground nutmeg

□ Preheat oven to 350°F. In small bowl, combine graham
cracker and bran flake crumbs, margarine and cinnamon;
spoon into 9-inch pie plate, pressing down firmly. Bake 8
to 10 minutes or until brown. Cool on wire rack.

In small saucepan, sprinkle gelatin over apple juice; set
aside 5 minutes or until gelatin softens. Over low heat,
cook, stirring constantly, 5 minutes or until gelatin dissolves; pour into large bowl.

In blender or food processor, puree 2 cups peaches; stir in gelatin. Add to bowl with yogurt, sugar, vanilla and nutmeg; stir until smooth. Cover and refrigerate 40 minutes or until mixture mounds when dropped from a spoon.

Coarsely chop remaining peaches; fold into gelatin mixture. Spoon into pie crust and refrigerate until firm. **MAKES 8 SERVINGS.**

APPROXIMATE NUTRIENT ANALYSIS PER SERVING:

Calories □ 190
Protein □ 5 grams
Fat □ 7 grams
Carbohydrate □ 30 grams
Cholesterol □ 3 milligrams
Sodium □ 170 milligrams
Potassium □ 335 milligrams

% Calories from Fat □ 30
% Calories from Saturated Fat
   □ 7
% Calories from
  Monounsaturated Fat □ 12
% Calories from Polyunsaturated
  Fat □ 11
P/S □ 1.4

FOOD GROUP UNITS

Fruits □ 1
Grains □ 1

Fat:
  Polyunsaturated □ 1¼
Sugars □ ½

RICE PUDDING MOLD

2 envelopes unflavored gelatin
1 cup cold water, divided
2 cups warm skim milk
¼ cup sugar
2 teaspoons vanilla extract
1 teaspoon ground cinnamon

⅛ teaspoon ground allspice
⅛ teaspoon salt
2 cups cooked rice
½ cup nonfat dry milk
Fresh fruit (optional)

□ In small saucepan, sprinkle gelatin over ½ cup cold water; set aside 5 minutes or until gelatin softens. Over low heat cook, stirring occasionally, about 5 minutes or until gelatin dissolves. Pour mixture into large bowl; cool 5 minutes. Beat in warm milk, sugar, vanilla, cinnamon, allspice and salt; stir in rice. Cover and refrigerate 50 minutes or until mixture mounds slightly when dropped from a spoon.

In chilled bowl with chilled beaters, beat nonfat dry milk and remaining cold water until soft peaks form; fold into rice mixture. Spray 1½-quart mold with nonstick cooking spray. Spoon mixture into mold. Cover and refrigerate about 8 hours. Invert onto serving plate. Serve with fresh fruit (if desired). **MAKES 8 SERVINGS.**

APPROXIMATE NUTRIENT ANALYSIS PER SERVING:

Calories ◻ 125

Protein ◻ 6 grams

Fat ◻ 0

Carbohydrate ◻ 24 grams

Cholesterol ◻ 2 milligrams

Sodium ◻ 90 milligrams

Potassium ◻ 235 milligrams

% Calories from Fat ◻ 0

FOOD GROUP UNITS:

Grains ◻ 1½

PAVLOVA

3 egg whites, at room
    temperature
⅛ teaspoon cream of tartar
⅓ cup sugar
1 teaspoon vanilla extract,
    divided

½ cup nonfat dry milk
½ cup ice water
1½ cups fresh or frozen,
    thawed unsweetened
    strawberries, sliced
1 cup kiwi slices

◻ Preheat oven to 250°F. Line baking sheet with parchment or brown paper. Draw an 8-inch circle in center; set aside.

In large bowl with mixer at high speed, beat egg whites and cream of tartar until soft peaks form; gradually add sugar and ½ teaspoon vanilla. Spoon meringue in center of circle on baking sheet; spread to edge of circle, forming 1½-inch rim. Bake 1¼ hours or until firm. Turn off oven. Let meringue cool in oven 2 hours without opening door.

In chilled bowl with chilled beaters, beat nonfat dry milk, water and remaining vanilla until stiff peaks form; spread over meringue. Arrange strawberries and kiwi fruit over top. MAKES 8 SERVINGS.

APPROXIMATE NUTRIENT ANALYSIS PER SERVING:

Calories □ 75

% Calories from Fat □ 0

Protein □ 2 grams

Fat □ 0

Carbohydrate □ 17 grams

Cholesterol □ 0

Sodium □ 30 milligrams

Potassium □ 215 milligrams

FOOD GROUP UNITS:

Fruits □ 1½

Sugars □ ½

Meat and Alternatives:

Very Low-Fat □ ½

CHAPTER VI

□

ON YOUR OWN

□ By reading this book, you have already taken the first steps toward changing diet, behavior, and exercise patterns. These chapters will guide you on the path to living well. But following that path is up to you. Only you have the power to take charge and follow through on your new plan for better health.

Keep in mind the factors that increase risk for atherosclerosis and coronary heart disease in persons who, like you, have been diagnosed as having elevated cholesterol. Cigarette smoking, obesity, insufficient exercise, high blood pressure and diabetes all compound the danger of disease in a person who also has the major risk factor of high cholesterol. How fortunate that you can eliminate or control these risk factors by simply making the one-day-at-a-time choice to live a healthy life.

Millions of Americans have already made this choice, shifting toward vegetables, fruit, fish and chicken and away from the saturated fats found in meat, butter, lard, milk and cream. According to the U. S. Department of Agriculture, there has been a marked improvement in per capita consumption of products affecting coronary heart disease risks. Since 1960, use of eggs is down 21 percent, fluid milk and cream down 19 percent and butter down 43 percent.[11] Consumption of fish and chicken are up 20 percent, respectively.[12,13] Purchase of low-fat and skim-milk products has increased by 300 percent since 1970.[17]

Advice from the Framingham Heart Study, a recent epidemiologic study on heart disease and diet, states: "If Americans would smoke less, get more regular exercise, keep their weight normal, follow a diet lower in fats and take care of their blood pressure, they would have better chances of avoiding, or at least postponing, heart problems."[18]

Diet alone—monitoring intake of calories, cholesterol, fats and sodium—can go a long way in reducing the risk of atherosclerosis and coronary heart disease. For example, excess weight and high blood pressure go hand in hand. Besides controlling weight by reducing fluid retention, lowering sodium intake is an important step in controlling blood pressure.

Diabetes, another risk factor, may often be controlled by diet. Just losing weight will bring certain types of diabetes under control.

A healthful diet combined with exercise is doubly effective in helping to guard your health. Studies have shown that exercise alone helps keep cholesterol levels low.

For one study, Finnish lumberjacks consumed about 4,760 calories daily, with a high proportion of their fat obtained from animal sources. Yet their blood cholesterol levels were no higher than those of other men in the same area who ate less fat. The Finnish researchers believe that physical activity was an important factor in keeping cholesterol levels low.[19]

After receiving your doctor's approval, it is recommended that you begin your exercise program with walking. As soon as you get the medical okay, get started! You don't need trendy, expensive clothes; you don't need a team, an opponent or a partner; you don't need to drive anywhere, invest in equipment or join costly clubs. All you have to do is step out your front door to start on the path toward living healthfully.

Changing what you eat and increasing your exercise usually require special effort. In Chapter II, Dr. Foreyt showed you how to change your behavior to make this task easier. With behavior modification, you prepare yourself for dieting and give yourself the tools to stick to your new diet plan.

Just as it helps to talk to friends who are also changing their behavior, it can be beneficial to talk to yourself. Listen to what you are saying to yourself. Are you talking positively, helping yourself make changes in your behavior? Or are you saying negative things that will chip away at your determination and perseverance?

Remind yourself frequently that changing eating habits takes time. Review all the changes you have made so far, and pat yourself on the back. Dr. Foreyt's behavior-modification method, which rewards good behavior rather than punishing you when you slip up, puts you on the road to correcting ingrained eating habits that may be harmful to your health.

The Beginning

This book has shown you how to guard your heart health by paying attention to two things: diet and exercise. By following a sensible, nutritionally balanced diet, you can control your weight. By establishing a regular exercise program, you can strengthen and tone your body. At the same time, you will burn calories at a more rapid rate, making your weight-control task easier. Finally, by following the behavior-modification program outlined in this book, you give yourself the tools needed to fit your diet and exercise into your daily life for better health the rest of your life.

If something is wrong with your car, you fix it. Why not do the same for yourself?

Cholesterol Content in Foods*

FOOD GROUP UNITS	LOW (0–25 mg)	MEDIUM (26–50 mg)	HIGH (50+ mg)
Vegetables	All		
Fruits	All		
Grains	Bread, sandwich	Egg noodles	
	Bread sticks		
	Cereal, dry and hot		
	Graham crackers		
	English muffins		
	Pasta and noodles (non-egg based)		
	Rice		
	Rolls, soft and hard		

*Based on commonly eaten portion sizes, with data obtained from *Bowes & Church's Food Values of Portions Commonly Used,* by Jean A. Pennington and Helen Nicholas Church, Philadelphia, J. B. Lippincott Company, 1980.

FOOD GROUP UNITS	LOW	MEDIUM	HIGH
Legumes	All		
Meats and Alternatives	Chicken, without skin Peanut butter Luncheon meats Cheese spreads Cheese food products	Cheese, hard (1 ounce) Cottage cheese, creamed Chicken, with skin Fish, except shrimp	Lamb Beef Pork Shrimp Eggs Organ meats
Milk Products	Evaporated milk, skim or low-fat Skim milk Yogurt, plain (skim and low-fat) Low-fat milk, 1% and 2%		
Fats	Margarine Mayonnaise Salad dressing, except cheese-based		Butter Lard

Types of Fats in Common Fat Products*

High in Polyunsaturates

Hollywood® safflower oil
Sunflower oil
Mazola® corn oil
Cottonseed oil
Tub margarine, made with safflower oil (regular and unsalted)
Sesame seed oil
Mayonnaise
Salad dressing, without cheese

High in Monounsaturates

Olive oil
Puritan® canola oil or rapeseed oil
Partially hydrogenated vegetable shortening
Peanut oil
Stick margarines, made with partially hydrogenated oil (regular and unsalted)
Imitation margarine

*Products are listed from highest to lowest content of fat type in each category.

High in Saturates	*High in Saturates & Cholesterol*
Crisco®	Butter
hydrogenated	Lard
shortening	Beef fat
Coconut oil	
Palm-kernel oil	
Palm oil	
Bacon drippings	
Meat drippings	

APPENDIX C

□

Sodium Content in Foods*

FOOD GROUP UNITS	LOW (0–100 mg)	MEDIUM (101–500 mg)	HIGH (500 + mg)
Vegetables	All, except canned and frozen	Canned and frozen	
Fruits	All		
Grains	Cereal, dry	Bread sticks	
	Graham crackers	Bread,	
	Pasta and noodles	sandwich	
	Rice	Rolls, soft and hard	
		Cereal, hot	
		English muffins	
		Muffins	
		Cornbread	
Legumes	All, except canned	Canned	

*Based on commonly eaten portion sizes, with data obtained from *Bowes & Church's Food Values of Portions Commonly Used,* by Jean A. Pennington and Helen Nicholas Church, Philadelphia, J. B. Lippincott Company, 1980.

FOOD GROUP UNITS	LOW	MEDIUM	HIGH
Meats and Alternatives	Organ meats Eggs Fish, including shellfish Chicken, with and without skin Turkey, with and without skin Beef, except canned, frozen and dried	Pork Peanut butter Cheese, hard Luncheon meats Cheese-food products	Cottage cheese Tuna, packed in oil or water Beef, canned, frozen, and dried
Milk Products		Evaporated milk, skim or low-fat Low-fat milk, 1% and 2% Skim milk Yogurt, plain (skim and low-fat)	
Fats	Mayonnaise Margarine Salad dressings	Lard Butter	

APPENDIX D

☐

Omega-3 Fatty Acid Composition of Various Fish*

LOW	MEDIUM	HIGH
(0.5 grams and under)	(0.6 to 1.0 grams)	(More than 1.0 gram)
Sole	Channel catfish	Rainbow trout
Northern pike	Red snapper	Cisco
Pacific cod	Yellowfin tuna	Pacific mackerel
Atlantic cod	Turbot	Atlantic herring
Walleye	Thread herring	Pacific herring
Yellow perch	Chum salmon	Sardine
Haddock	Striped bass	American eel
Yellowtail	Wolffish	Atlantic halibut
Sturgeon	Spot	Sablefish
Rockfish	Swordfish	Atlantic salmon
Brook trout		Lake trout
Silver hake		Anchovy
Striped mullet		Coho salmon
Atlantic pollock		Pink salmon

*Based on data obtained from the United States Department of Agriculture. Values are for 100 grams of fish.

LOW	MEDIUM	HIGH
Ocean perch		Bluefin tuna
Carp		Atlantic mackerel
Pacific halibut		King salmon
Pacific whiting		Spiny dogfish
Weakfish		Albacore tuna
Skipjack tuna		Sockeye salmon

NOTES

[1] The Lipid Research Clinics Coronary Primary Prevention Trial Results: I, "Reduction in Incidence of Coronary Heart Disease," *Journal of the American Medical Association 251* (1984): 351.

[2] The Lipid Research Clinics Coronary Primary Prevention Trial Results: II, "The Relationship of Reduction in Incidence of Coronary Heart Disease to Cholesterol Lowering," *Journal of the American Medical Association 251* (1984): 365.

[3] American Heart Association, "Risk Factors and Coronary Disease: A Statement for Physicians," *Circulation 62* (1980): 445A–451A.

[4] F. Grande et al, "Sucrose and Various Carbohydrate-Containing Foods and Serum Lipids in Man," *American Journal of Clinical Nutrition 27* (1974): 1043–1051.

[5] D. L. Robertson et al, "Epidemiologic Studies of Coronary Heart Disease and Stroke in Japanese Men in Japan, Hawaii and California. Coronary Heart Disease Risk Factors in Japan and Hawaii," *American Journal of Cardiology 39* (1977): 244–249.

[6] Multiple Risk Factor Intervention Trial Research Group, "Multiple Risk Factor Intervention Trial: Risk Factor Changes and Mortality Results," *Journal of the American Medical Association 248* (1982): 1465–1477.

[7] H. O. Bang et al, "The Composition of the Eskimo Food in Northwestern Greenland," *American Journal of Clinical Nutrition 33* (1980): 2657–2661.

[8]D. Kromhout et al, "The Inverse Relation between Fish Consumption and 20-Year Mortality from Coronary Heart Disease," *New England Journal of Medicine 312* (1985): 1205–1209.

[9]S. M. Grundy, "Comparison of Monounsaturated Fatty Acids and Carbohydrates for Lowering Plasma Cholesterol," *New England Journal of Medicine 314* (1986): 745.

[10]J. W. Anderson et al, "Hypocholesterolemic Effects of Oat Bran or Bean Intake for Hypercholesterolemic Men," *American Journal of Clinical Nutrition 40* (1984): 1146–1155.

[11]U.S. Department of Agriculture Economic Research Service, "Food Consumption, Prices and Expenditures," *Statistical Bulletin*, (September 1981), pp. 127, 671, 672.

[12]U.S. Department of Commerce, *Statistical Abstract of the U.S., 1982–1983*. (Washington, D.C.: U.S. Government Printing Office, 1983) p. 706.

[13]Commodity Research Bureau, Inc., *Commodity Year Book, 1983*, (May 1983), p. 65.

[14]U.S. Department of Health and Human Services, USDA, *Nutrition Monitoring in the United States—A Progress Report from the Joint Nutrition Monitoring Evaluation Committee*, (July 1986), p. 77.

[15]General Mills, *A Status Report on the American Diet and Health—1980*. (Minneapolis: General Mills Nutrition Department, 1980), pp. 7–8.

[16]American Heart Association, "Dietary Guidelines for Healthy American Adults: A Statement for Physicians and Health Professionals by the Nutrition Committee, American Heart Association," *Circulation 74* (1986): 1465A–1468A.

[17]B. Peterkin et al, "Food Patterns—Where Are We Headed?" *Food from Farm to Table, 1982 Year Book of Agriculture.* (Washington, D.C.: U.S. Government Printing Office, 1982), p. 230.

[18]W. McDade, "Good News from the House on Lincoln Street," *Fortune,* January 14, 1982, pp. 86–92.

[19]"Diet and Serum Cholesterol Levels of Lumberjacks," *Nutrition Reviews 20* (1962): 4–5.

I N D E X   O F   R E C I P E S
(nutritional information follows each recipe)

215

ABOUT THE AUTHOR

GAIL BECKER, a registered dietitian, earned her degree in dietetics from Drexel University. She has managed the food and nutrition department of the world's largest weight-control organization, directed dietetics at a large metropolitan hospital and headed dietetic services for a major food company. Ms. Becker currently serves on the Subcommittee on Nutrition Program of the American Heart Association, the Society for Nutrition Education, American College of Nutrition, the Institute of Food Technology, the American Home Economics Association and many other professional organizations. She conducts nutrition seminars and appears frequently on television and radio programs as an authority on nutrition. Her published articles have appeared in leading women's magazines.

Ms. Becker is the president of a Great Neck, New York-based public relations/marketing communications company serving the food, nutrition and health-promotion industries.